MOOD FOOD

MOOD FOOD

CHEF AND CO-WRITER ROB MURRAY
CO-WRITER/ART DIRECTOR/EDITOR/PHOTOGRAPHER NIKI MURRAY
GRAPHIC DESIGNER MEGAN BEDFORD

First Edition, 2021
Published by Nice to Meet You LLC

Copyright © 2021 Nice to Meet You LLC

Mention of specific companies, organizations, or authorities in this book does not imply endorsement by the author or publisher, nor does mention of specific companies, organizations, or authorities imply that they endorse this book, its author, or the publisher.

All content contained in this book is for information purposes only. The information in this book is not a substitute for professional medical advice, diagnosis or treatment.

All rights reserved.

Without limiting the rights under the copyright reserved above, no part of this publication may be reproduced, stored in, or introduced into a retrieval system, or transmitted, in any form, or by any means (electrical, mechanical, photocopying, recording, or otherwise) without the prior written permission of the copyright owner.

Library of Congress Catalog Number 2021922742
ISBN-13: 979-8-9852486-1-6

All photographs copyright © Niki Murray

WWW.MOODFOODCOOKBOOK.COM

EAT YOUR FEELINGS,

MOOD FOOD

EMBRACE YOUR LIFE

BY NIKI & ROB MURRAY

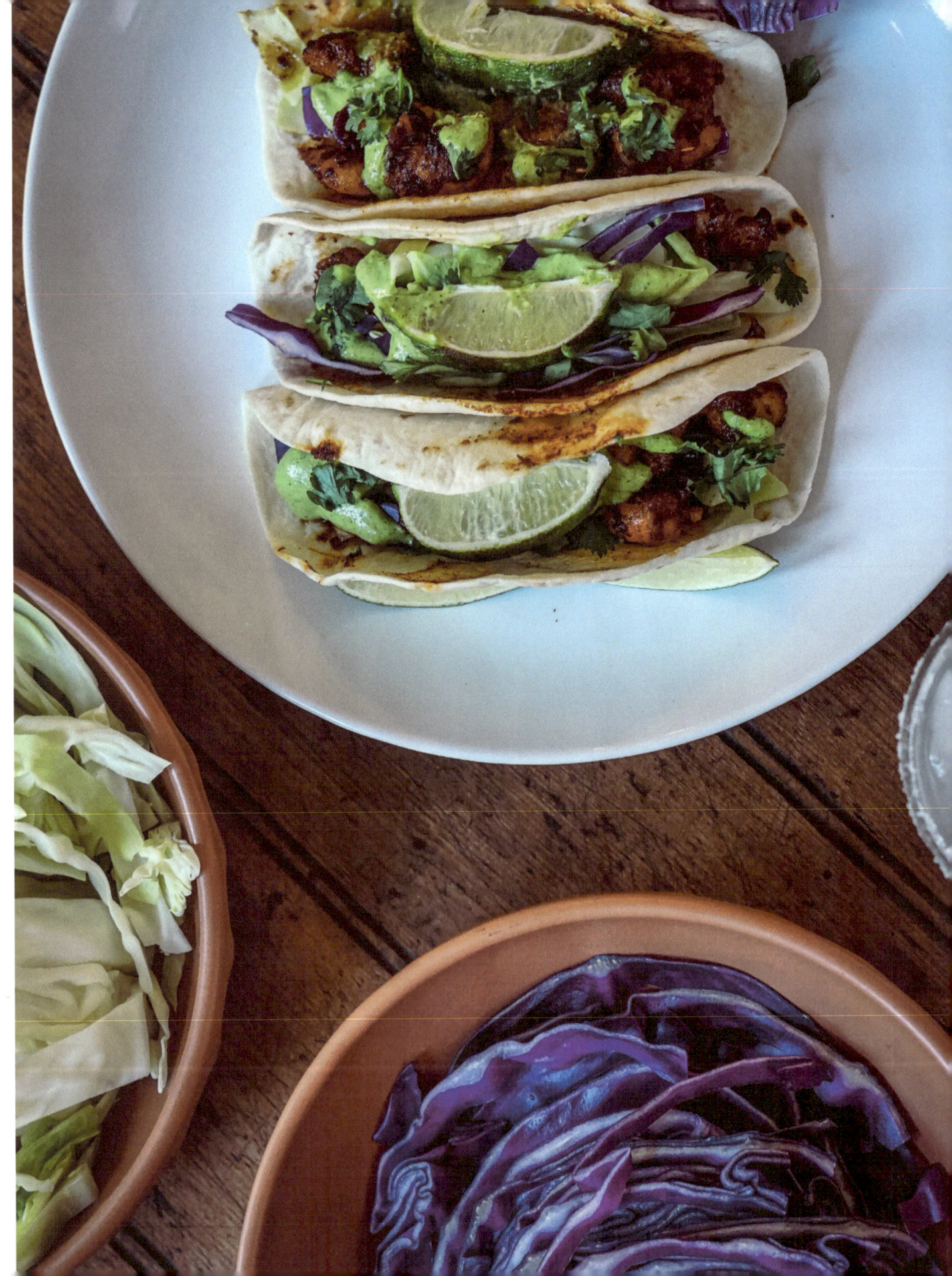

Dedicated to the folks that attended our "family" dinners,
didn't laugh at our idea for a mood-based cookbook,
and ate all the leftovers along the way.

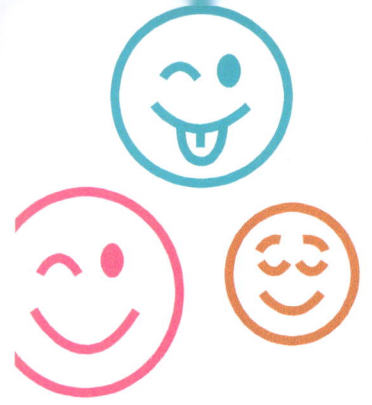

you deserve good food,
    whatever comes your way

no matter the mood,
    this is your chance to play

check in with your feelings

pick something on the right

we'll make it taste great

and everything will be alright

ADVENTUROUS
DARING | PLAYFUL | CURIOUS

BEAT
TIRED | OVERWHELMED | IN NEED OF A BOOST

BROKE
TAPPED | STRAPPED | SAVING

COZY
COLD | COUCHY | IN NEED OF A HUG

FLIRTY
FRISKY | SASSY | ROMANTIC

MYSELF
INDULGENT | CELEBRATORY | BOLD

PANICKED
STRESSED | RUSHED | ENTERTAINING

SPORTY
MUNCHY | PUNCHY | CHEERFUL

TABLE OF CONTENTS

FEELING ADVENTUROUS — 1

- KOREAN PULLED PORK SANDWICH — 3
- SPICY TUNA BITES — 5
- SAUSAGE ROLLS — 7
- SWEET ONION CHUTNEY — 9
- TOM YUM(MY) SOUP — 10
- EGGS IN PURGATORY — 11
- PEANUT CURRY — 13
- TANDOORI-LESS CHICKEN — 15
- SHORT ORDER CHICKEN — 17
- THAI LAAB SALAD — 19
- POBLANO PALOMA — 20
- WHITE NEGRONI — 21
- PINEAPPLE TURMERIC MARGARITA — 22

FEELING BEAT — 23

- CHEAT CODE CHILAQUILES — 25
- ROTISSERIE CHICKEN NOODLE SOUP — 26
- PEANUTTY PASTA & BLANCHED KALE — 27
- INSTANT ENERGY KALE SALAD — 29
- TATOR TOT HOT DISH — 30
- EASY CARAMEL APPLE DIP — 31
- SIMPLE SHRIMP & AVOCADO BITES — 32

FEELING BROKE — 33

- RENT CONTROL RAMEN — 35
- SOY CHEAP EGGS — 36
- CASH-STRAPPED CAULIFLOWER STEAKS — 37
- CHOCOLATE DROP COOKIES — 39
- GRANDMA NIXA'S BUNS — 40
- BUDGET BRUSCHETTA — 41
- PUDDING MYSELF THROUGH COLLEGE PIE — 42
- PIZZA DOUGH — 43
- RAMEN POPCORN — 45
- GOLD RUSH — 46

FEELING COZY — 47

- SLOW MORNING MONKEY BREAD — 49
- PANCAKES + CINNAMON HASH — 51
- FRENCH ONION SOUP — 53
- CHICKEN POCKET PIES — 55
- COMFY CORNBREAD CASSEROLE — 57
- GRANDMA MURRAY'S BEEF STEW — 59
- SPECIAL K BARS — 60
- TOMATO SOUP + GRILLED CHEESE — 61
- CHEDDAR BISCUITS + GRAVY — 63
- MELLOW MASH — 65
- PENICILLIN — 66
- CLASSIC OLD FASHIONED — 67
- CAMPFIRE OLD FASHIONED — 68

FEELING FLIRTY — 69

- TANTALIZING TIRAMISU — 71
- MY PLACE PORKETTA — 73
- SWEETHEART-WORTHY STUFFED SHELLS — 75
- RASPBERRY + WHITE CHOCOLATE MUFFINS — 77
- BOTH WAYS DEVILED EGGS — 79
- ROASTED RED PEPPER SALMON — 81
- FRENCH SILK PIE — 83
- SEARED SCALLOPS + GNOCCHI — 85
- SMOKESHOW SALMON BENEDICT — 87
- NEW YORK SOUR — 89
- PAPER PLANES — 90

FEELING MYSELF — 91

- SASSY SHRIMP TACOS — 93
- MY WAY MAC + CHEESE — 95
- SEA SALT + CHOCOLATE CHIP COOKIES — 97
- SALMON CROQUETTES — 99
- CRUNKWRAPS — 101
- CHEDDAR SCALLION SCONES — 103
- MARRY MYSELF CHICKEN — 105
- BREAKFAST BFFS — 107

TABLE OF CONTENTS

FEELING MYSELF (CONTINUED)

BITCHIN' BIRTHDAY CAKE	109
BOURBON BUBBLE SUGAR	111
MULLED CIDER	112
BEES KNEES	113
GOOD DAY GRASSHOPPER	114

FEELING PANICKED — 115

GOAT CHEESE + APRICOT CROSTINI	117
WARP SPEED SALSA DIP	118
EASY AFRICAN PEANUT SOUP	119
CUTE LITTLE PINEAPPLE CAKES	121
PAN FRIED GNOCCHI	123
SPEEDY GRILLED SHRIMP	125
AROMATIC ROASTED GARLIC	126
ROASTED GARLIC PULL-APART BREAD	127
SNAPPY AVOCADO + SHRIMP TOAST	129
SLAP-IT-TOGETHER SANGRIA	130
FRENCH 75	131
BLACK CAULDRON	132

FEELING SPORTY — 133

CRISPY BAKED CHICKEN WINGS	135
SMASH BURGERS + SAUCE	137
WINNING STREAK SMASHED POTATOES	138
BUFFALO CHEESE DIP	139
PARTY-WORTHY PESTO	140
(ALMOST) CUBAN SLIDERS	141
MVP BEER PUNCH	143

INDEX	145
ABOUT THE AUTHORS	148

ALLERGY GUIDE

HERE'S THE DEAL

Mood Food recipes can be modified to fit your allergies, dietary restrictions, or preferences. Some recipes are naturally gluten-free, dairy-free, or vegan.

A QUICK GUIDE TO THE LABELS ON EACH PAGE:

- **GF** This recipe is gluten-free.
- **GF** This recipe can be made gluten-free with simple eliminations or substitutions.
- **DF** This recipe is dairy-free.
- **DF** This recipe can be made dairy-free with simple eliminations or substitutions.
- **V** This recipe is vegan.
- **V** This recipe can be made vegan with simple eliminations or substitutions.

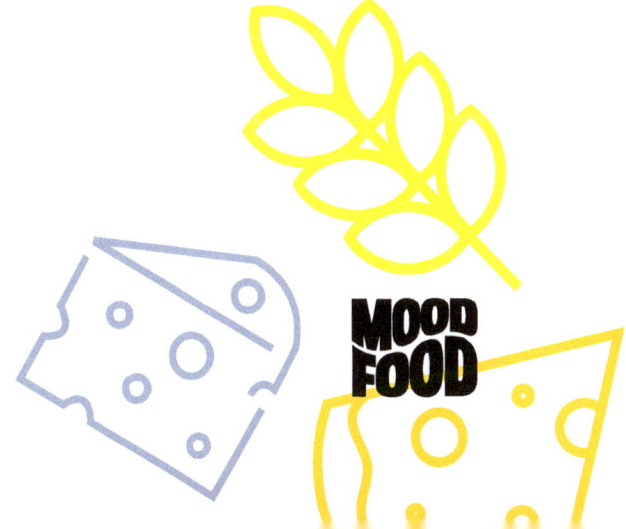

FEELING

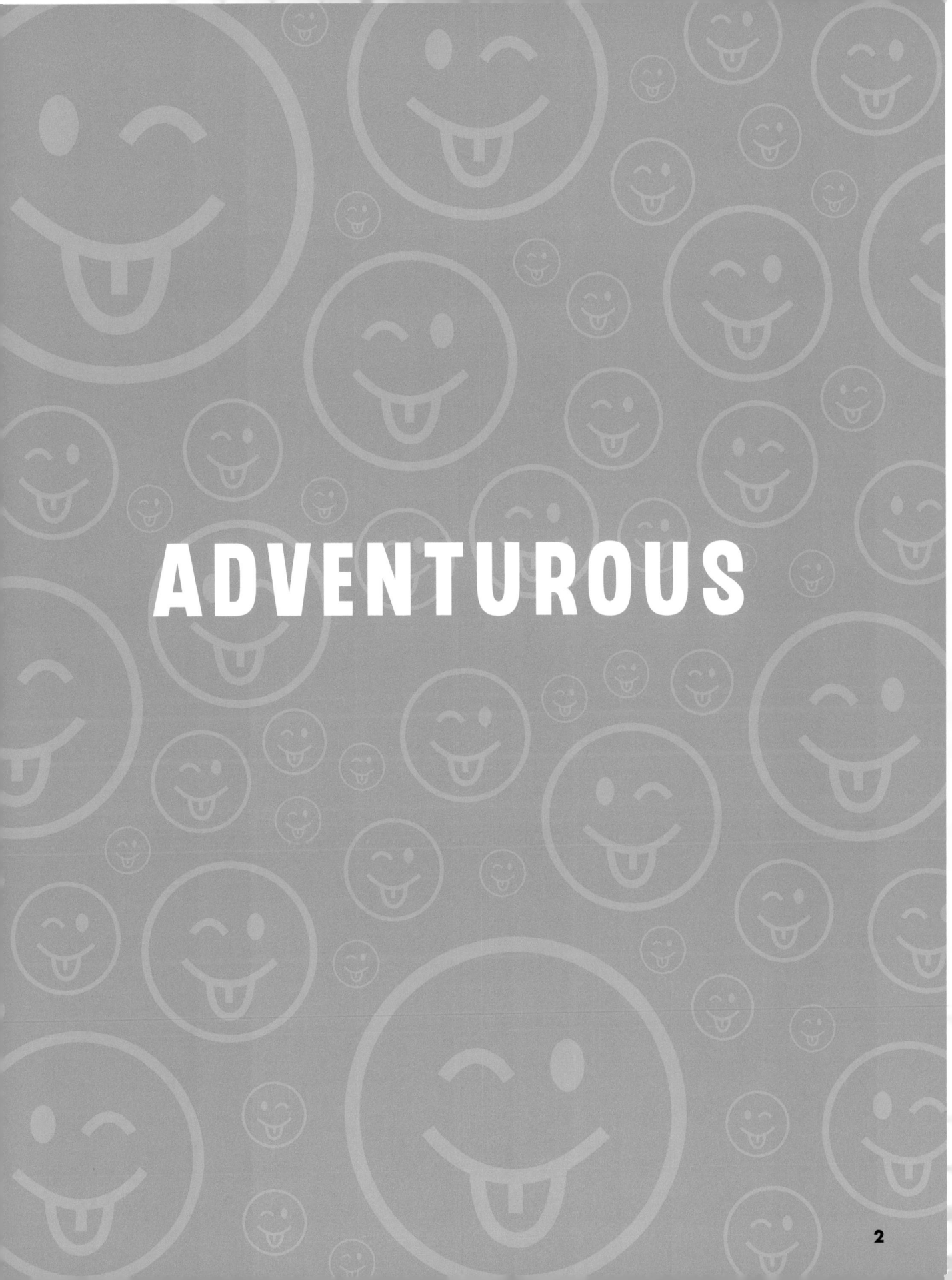
ADVENTUROUS

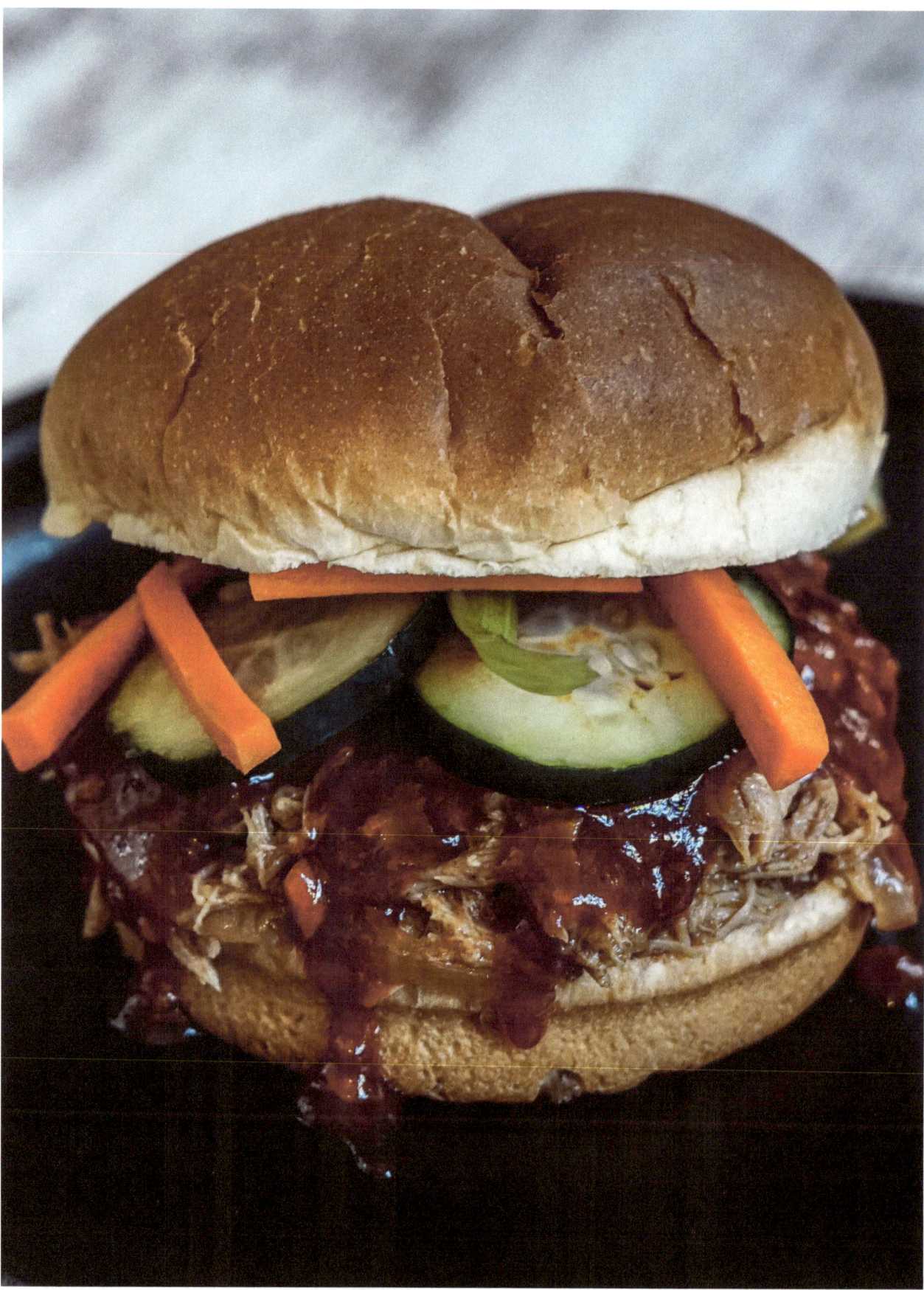

FEELING ADVENTUROUS

KOREAN PULLED PORK SANDWICH

MAKES 8 SAUCY SANDWICHES

PAIRS WELL WITH:
- THE NEED FOR NOVELTY
- CLOTHING YOU DON'T CARE ABOUT
- UPSTAGING GRANDMA AT THE FAMILY BBQ

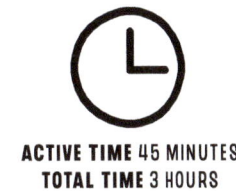

ACTIVE TIME 45 MINUTES
TOTAL TIME 3 HOURS

INGREDIENTS

PORK

4-6 pound pork shoulder (4 no-bone, 6 bone-in)
2 Tablespoons olive oil
2 large white onions, thinly sliced
1 cup chicken broth
3 Tablespoons gochujang (Korean chili paste)
3 Tablespoons rice vinegar
1 Tablespoon sesame oil
1 ½ Tablespoons garlic, minced
1 teaspoon salt
½ teaspoon pepper
8 hamburger buns

KOREAN BBQ SAUCE

3 Tablespoons gochujang
½ cup ketchup
¼ cup rice vinegar
¼ cup brown sugar
2 Tablespoons soy sauce
2 Tablespoons honey
4 cloves garlic, minced

PICKLED VEGGIES

2 Tablespoons sugar
¼ cup rice vinegar
1 cucumber, sliced
1 carrot, sliced into matchsticks
1 celery stalk, sliced into matchsticks

BACK TO BASICS

In the mood for a more traditional BBQ sandwich? Swap the gochujang for dijon mustard, the rice vinegar for apple cider vinegar, and ditch the sesame oil. Top with your favorite BBQ sauce and you're good to go.

INSTRUCTIONS

COOK THE PORK

Preheat the oven to 350°F. Place a rack on the lower third of the oven, low enough that you can easily put a stock pot on the bottom rack and close the door.

Cut the pork into 1 ½ inch chunks and season generously with salt and pepper. Heat olive oil in a stock pot on medium-high heat.

Slowly add the pork chunks to the pot, using batches to ensure you can brown each piece on all sides (if there's too much meat in the pot at once, the excess moisture will prevent it from browning properly).

In a separate bowl, combine the thinly sliced onion, chicken broth, gochujang, rice vinegar, sesame oil, garlic, salt and pepper, then add the mixture to the stock pot and stir until evenly distributed among the pork chunks.

Cover the pot (a lid or foil will do) and transfer to the oven. Bake for two hours or until the internal temperature of the pork reaches 145°F.

MAKE THE KOREAN BBQ SAUCE

In a small saucepan, combine all the ingredients and whisk over medium heat, bringing to a simmer. Once simmering, reduce to low and cook for 10 minutes. Remove from heat and let cool.

PICKLE THOSE VEGGIES

Mix sugar and vinegar in a bowl until sugar is dissolved, then pour over fresh vegetables and toss. If you're making this well in advance, we suggest you cover and refrigerate the veggies until you're ready to assemble sandwiches.

Remove the pork from the oven and use two forks to shred or "pull" the pork. Serve hot with pickled veggies and korean BBQ sauce!

TRAVEL TIP

Need to transport the pork to another location? After shredding, transfer to a slow cooker, then heat on low until ready to serve.

FEELING ADVENTUROUS

SPICY TUNA BITES

MAKES 80 BITES

PAIRS WELL WITH:
- SUSHI CRAVINGS (WITHOUT THE SUSHI ROLLING SKILLS)
- FRIENDS WHO NEVER EAT THE LAST BITE
- STARTING SMALL

TOTAL TIME 20 MINUTES

SPECIAL EQUIPMENT

Sharp knife
Large plate, platter, or cutting board
Squeeze bottle or sandwich bag (optional)

INGREDIENTS

½ cup mayo
1 Tablespoon sriracha
8 ounces sushi grade Ahi tuna, diced
⅓ cup teriyaki sauce
1 Tablespoon soy sauce
1 ½ teaspoons toasted sesame oil
2 cucumbers, sliced
2 avocados, thinly sliced
2 stalks green onion, diced (for garnish)
Black sesame seeds (for garnish)

INSTRUCTIONS

Mix the mayo and sriracha in a bowl, transfer to a sandwich bag or squeeze bottle, and set aside.

In a medium bowl, combine the tuna, teriyaki sauce, soy sauce, and sesame oil.

Cover and set aside.

Cut the cucumber into slices thick enough to stay rigid as you lift them to your mouth, then lay them out onto a large platter or plate.

Layer a spoonful of teriyaki tuna, an avocado slice, and squeeze of spicy mayo onto each slice.

Top with a sprinkling of green onion and sesame seeds and serve!

PRO TIP

If you put the spicy mayo into a bag, clip a small corner off with a pair of scissors, then squeeze a little mayo onto each piece.

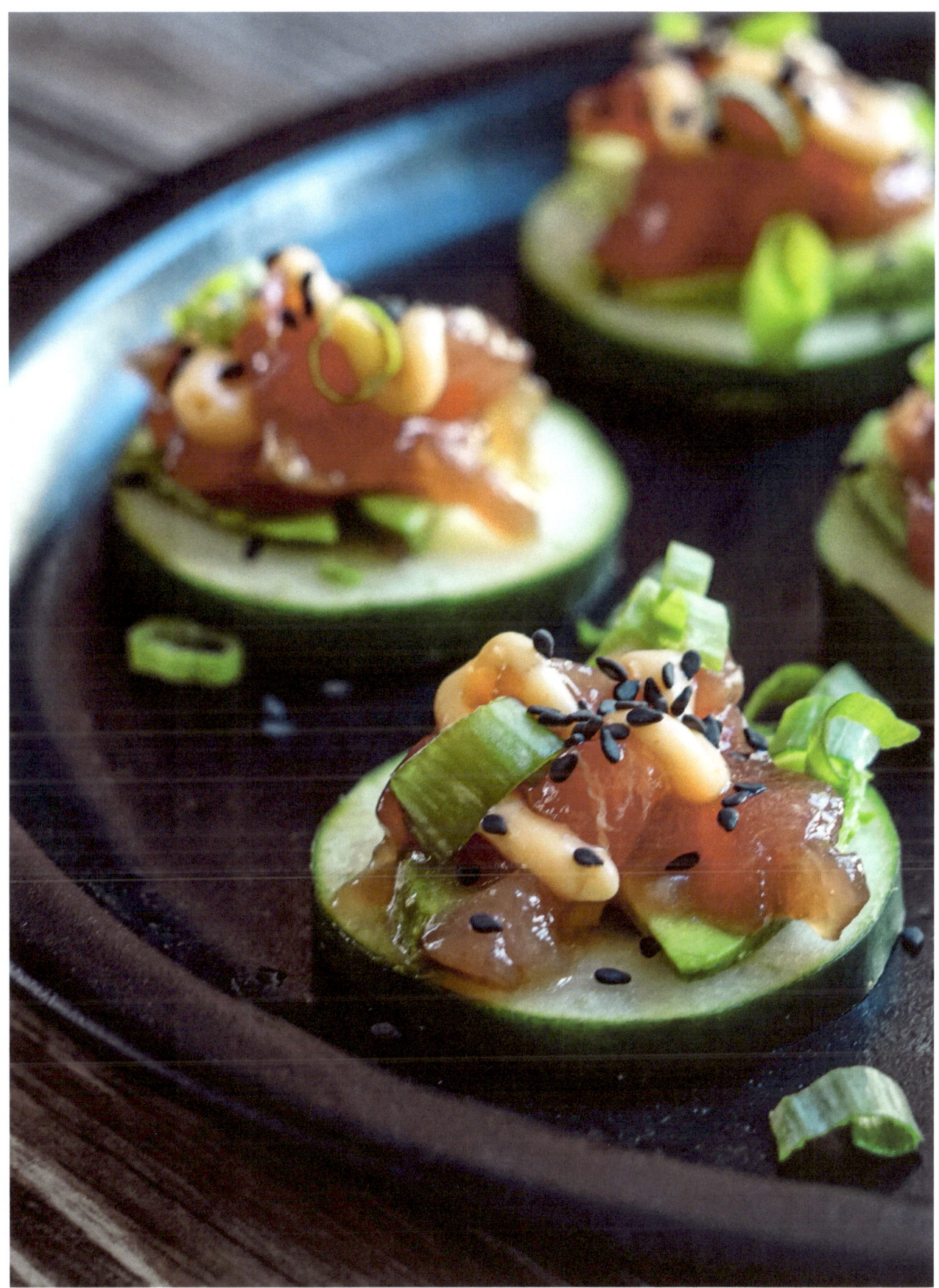

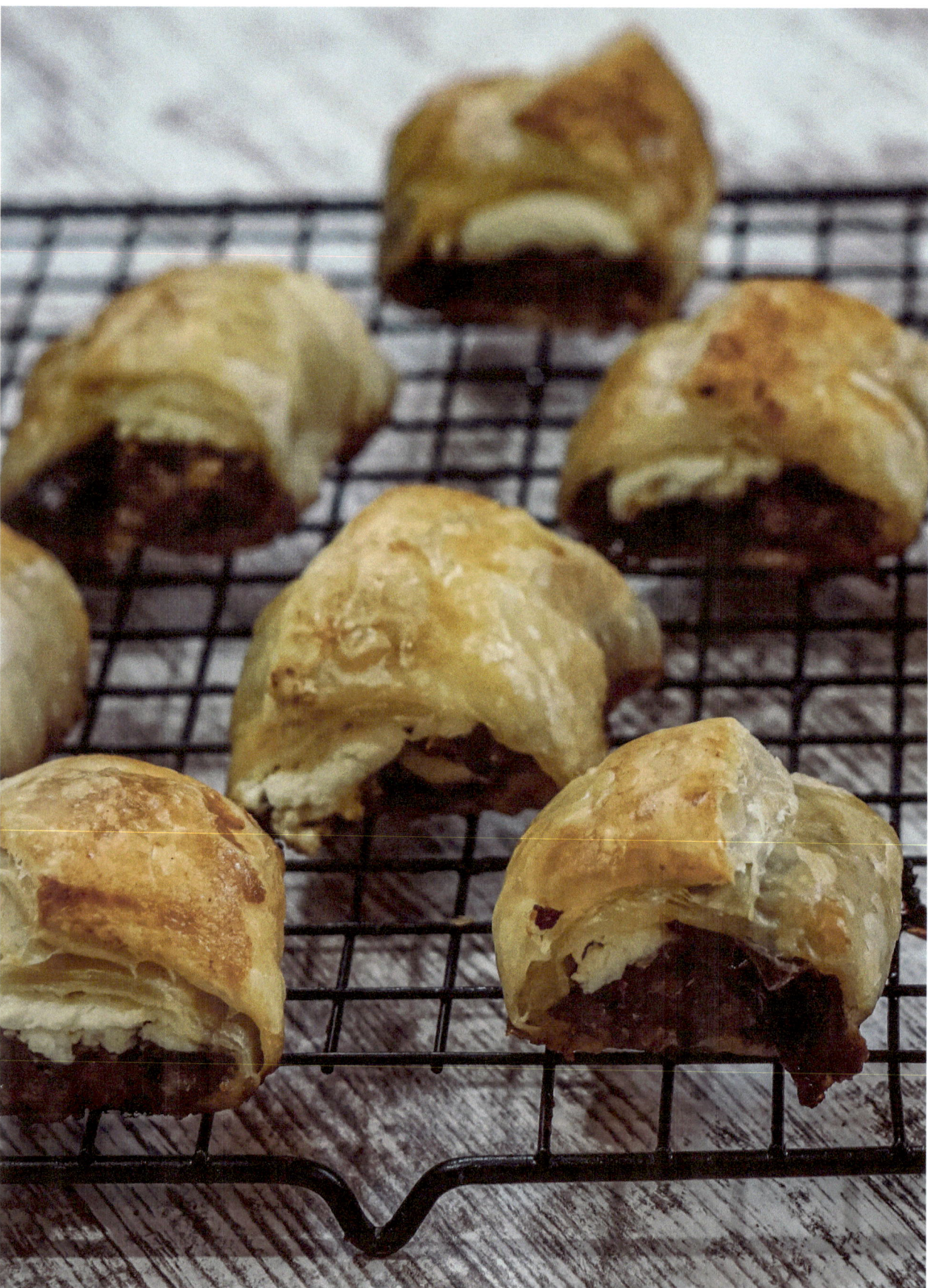

FEELING ADVENTUROUS

SAUSAGE ROLLS

MAKES 20 MINI-ROLLS
(ABOUT 5 SERVINGS)

PAIRS WELL WITH:
- BAD BRITISH ACCENTS
- FINGER FOOD AFICIONADOS
- SWEET ONION CHUTNEY (NEXT PAGE)

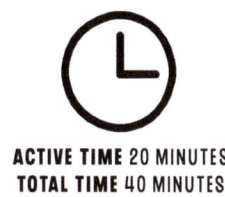

ACTIVE TIME 20 MINUTES
TOTAL TIME 40 MINUTES

FAIR WARNINGS

If you buy frozen puff pastry, you'll need to thaw it before starting this recipe!

If you decide to make the onion chutney on the next page, we suggest doing it in advance.

INGREDIENTS

2 sheets pre-made puff pastry
1 pound italian sausage
4 sprigs fresh (or 2 Tablespoons dried) sage, finely chopped
Sweet onion chutney
8 ounces soft goat cheese
1 egg

SERVE WITH

Onion chutney

INSTRUCTIONS

Preheat the oven to 400°F.

Unroll the thawed puff pastry onto a cutting board, then split it in half, lengthwise.

Place parchment paper on a baking sheet and set it aside.

In a medium mixing bowl, combine the sausage and sage with your hands until it makes gross sounds.

Spoon some chutney (or other sauce of choice) along the center of each pastry piece, then layer on the goat cheese every half-inch or so. We recommend leaving a little pastry exposed on the edges to help contain the filling.

Split the sausage mixture into two equal portions. Roll each one to the length of the pastry then lay it down the center.

Beat the egg in a small bowl, then use a brush or your fingers to "paint" the edges of the pastry. This will help the pastry stick to itself when you roll it up.

Roll the edges, one over the other until the sausage is completely wrapped. Brush the top of the roll with the egg again. For some reason, shiny dough tastes better.

With a sharp knife, cut each roll into bite-sized pieces and place it on the baking sheet.

Bake until golden brown (about 20 minutes).

Serve with more onion chutney (or another sauce of your choice) and enjoy!

FEELING ADVENTUROUS
SWEET ONION CHUTNEY

MAKES ABOUT 3 LARGE JARS

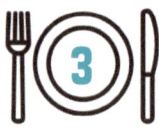

PAIRS WELL WITH:
- EVERYTHING. IT'S REALLY THAT GOOD.

ACTIVE TIME
45 MINUTES
TOTAL TIME
2 HOURS (IT'S WORTH IT)

SPECIAL EQUIPMENT
Ski goggles
(unless you need a good cry)

INGREDIENTS
- 3 Tablespoons olive oil
- 6 large red onions
- 1 large shallot
- 2 large white onions
- 1 - 3-inch cinnamon stick
- 2 bay leaves
- 1 sprig rosemary (leaves only), chopped
- 1 cup balsamic vinegar
- ¼ cup red wine vinegar
- 1 cup dark brown sugar

HERE'S THE DEAL
This chutney is delicious. This recipe will likely make more chutney than anyone (even you) can eat in one sitting. You can store it in the fridge, preserve it in a sterilized jar, or submit it to the State Fair. We won't tell.

INSTRUCTIONS
- Grab some ski goggles.
- Peel and chop onions and shallots.
- Put a large stock pot on medium-high heat, then add olive oil to the bottom of the pot.
- Once the oil has heated up, add onions, cinnamon, bay leaves, and rosemary.
- Turn heat to medium and cook until onions are soft and golden.
- Add the vinegar and sugar to the onions, then turn the heat down to low, stirring occasionally.
- Let the mixture meld for about an hour. Once it starts to thicken, you're good to go!

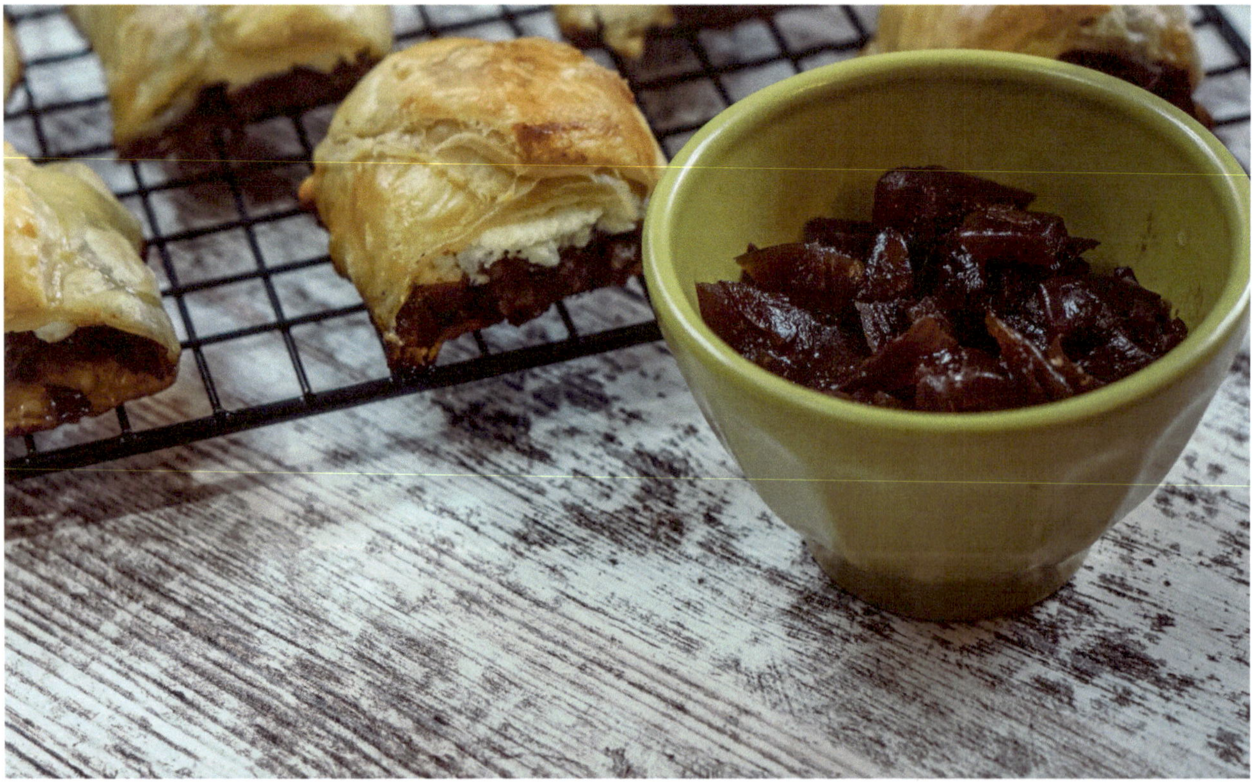

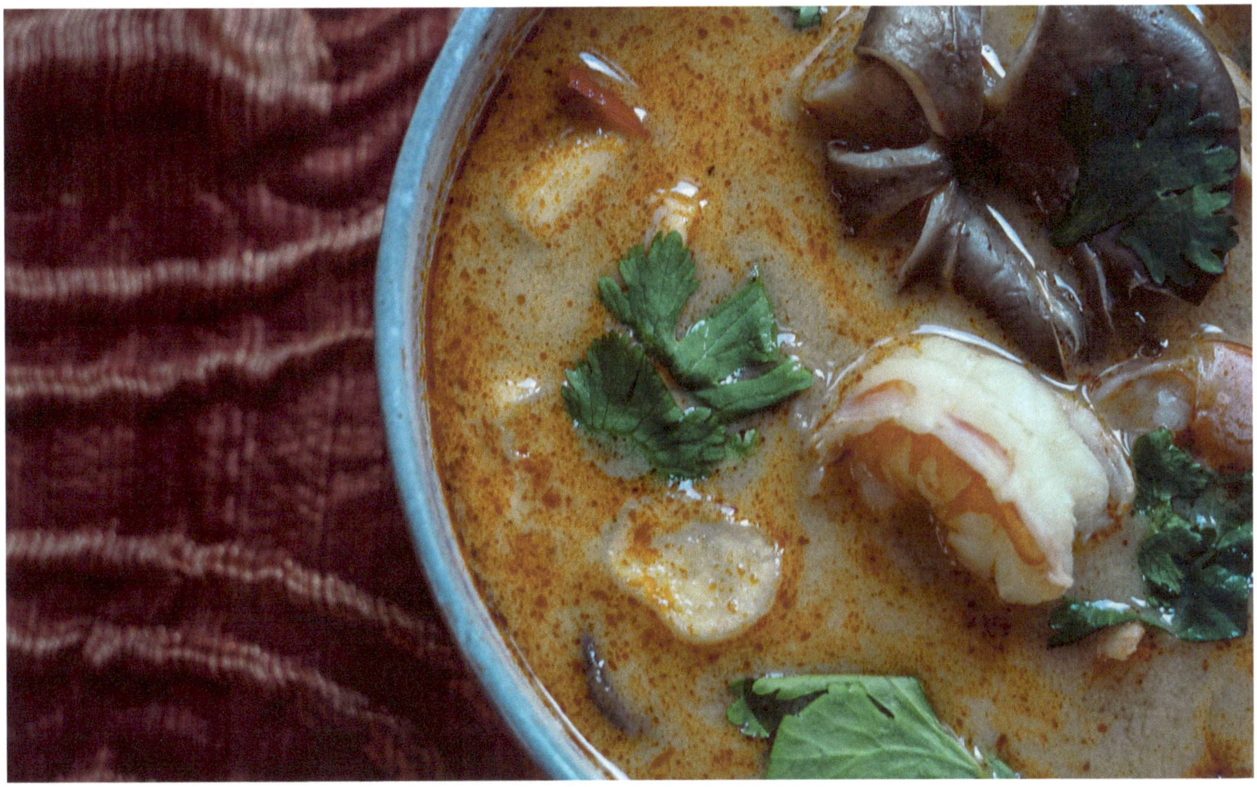

TOM YUM(MY) SOUP

MAKES 6-8 LARGE SERVINGS

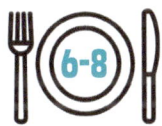

PAIRS WELL WITH:
- FRIENDS WHO LOVE SPICE
- HEAPS OF RICE
- FUNGI FREAKS

ACTIVE TIME
15 MINUTES
TOTAL TIME
30 MINUTES

INGREDIENTS
- Large shrimp (4-6 per person)
- 64 ounces chicken or veggie broth
- 2 Tablespoons Tom Yum paste (2T = medium heat)
- 1 clove garlic, minced
- ⅓ cup lemongrass (the white part), minced
- 5 lime leaves, crushed
- ⅓ cup fish sauce
- ½ cup coconut milk
- 1 cup oyster mushrooms, whole or sliced
- 3 Tablespoons lime juice

SERVE WITH
- Chili or Tom Yum paste
- Lime wedges
- Sugar
- Cilantro
- White rice

INSTRUCTIONS
- Start by shelling and deveining your shrimp. If you're using frozen and prepared shrimp, thaw in a large bowl with cold water for about 20 minutes.
- Once you've handled your shrimp, add the broth to a large pot and turn to medium-high. Add your Tom Yum paste, garlic, lemongrass, and lime leaves and get that shit to a rolling boil! When it starts boiling, turn the heat to medium and simmer for 10-15 minutes - we want those flavors to blend.
- After 10-15 minutes, add your fish sauce and coconut milk and simmer for a few minutes longer.
- Has it been a few minutes already? Nice - now add your shrimp and mushrooms and continue simmering for another three minutes.
- Once your shrimp is fully cooked (soft but not rubbery), add in the lime juice, give a quick stir and serve. You can ladle it into bowls by itself or stretch it a little by serving over rice.
- Serve with the above to adjust the flavors in real time and enjoy!

FEELING ADVENTUROUS

EGGS IN PURGATORY

MAKES 6 EGGS AND A HEAP OF SAUCE

PAIRS WELL WITH:
- FRIENDS WHO DON'T JUDGE YOU FOR LICKING THE PLATE
- SUNDAY MORNINGS
- CROONERS ON FULL BLAST

TOTAL TIME 30 MINUTES

SPECIAL EQUIPMENT

Deep-sided pan and lid
Large spoon for egg-scooping
Bread knife

INGREDIENTS

5 ounces pancetta
2 cloves garlic, minced
½ teaspoon crushed red pepper
2 cans (14.5 oz) diced fire-roasted or San Marzano tomatoes
6 eggs
Salt, to taste

SERVE WITH

Baguette, sliced
Basil
Olive oil

INSTRUCTIONS

Start by heating a large, deep-sided pan over medium-low heat.

Once the pan is warm, add the pancetta and let it cook for about five minutes.

Add the garlic and crushed red pepper and cook until you can smell it from your couch.

Turn the heat up to medium, then toss in the tomatoes.

Simmer, stirring occassionally, for about 10 minutes or until the tomatoes have broken down a bit and some of the tomatoey-water has evaporated, then turn the heat back down to medium-low.

With a spoon, create egg-sized depressions in the tomato mixture, one for each egg you're making (this can easily be done in two batches if you want to cook more than six eggs).

Crack an egg into each depression, put the lid on the pan, and cook the eggs for about six minutes. We like runny eggs for maximum bread-soppage, but feel free to go longer than six minutes if you prefer cooked yolks.

Once the eggs are cooked to your liking, remove the pan from heat and serve!

We like to garnish with basil, olive oil, and freshly cut baguette slices.

HOT TIP
Warm bread always tastes better, so we recommend popping the baguette in the oven or toaster right before serving.

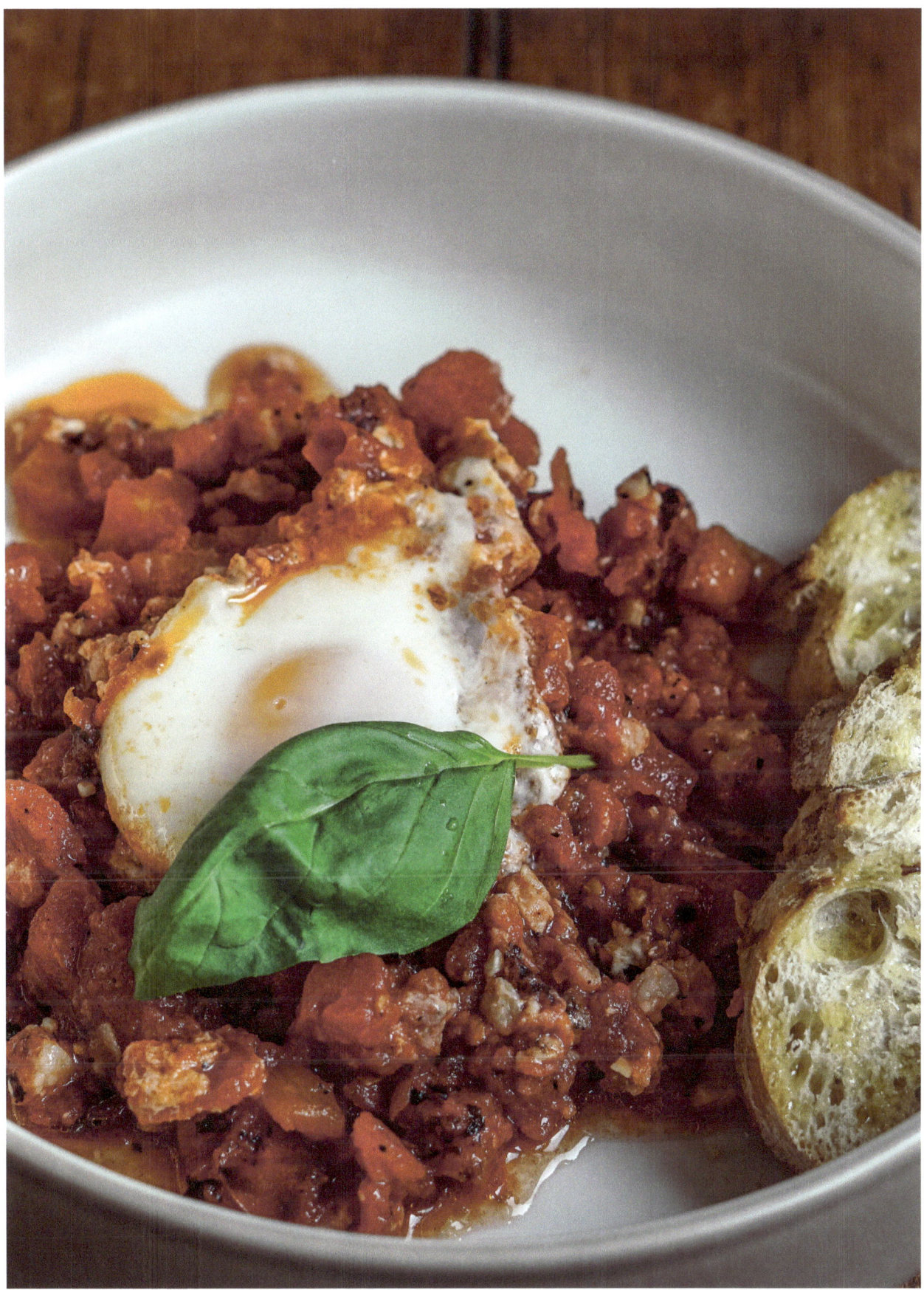

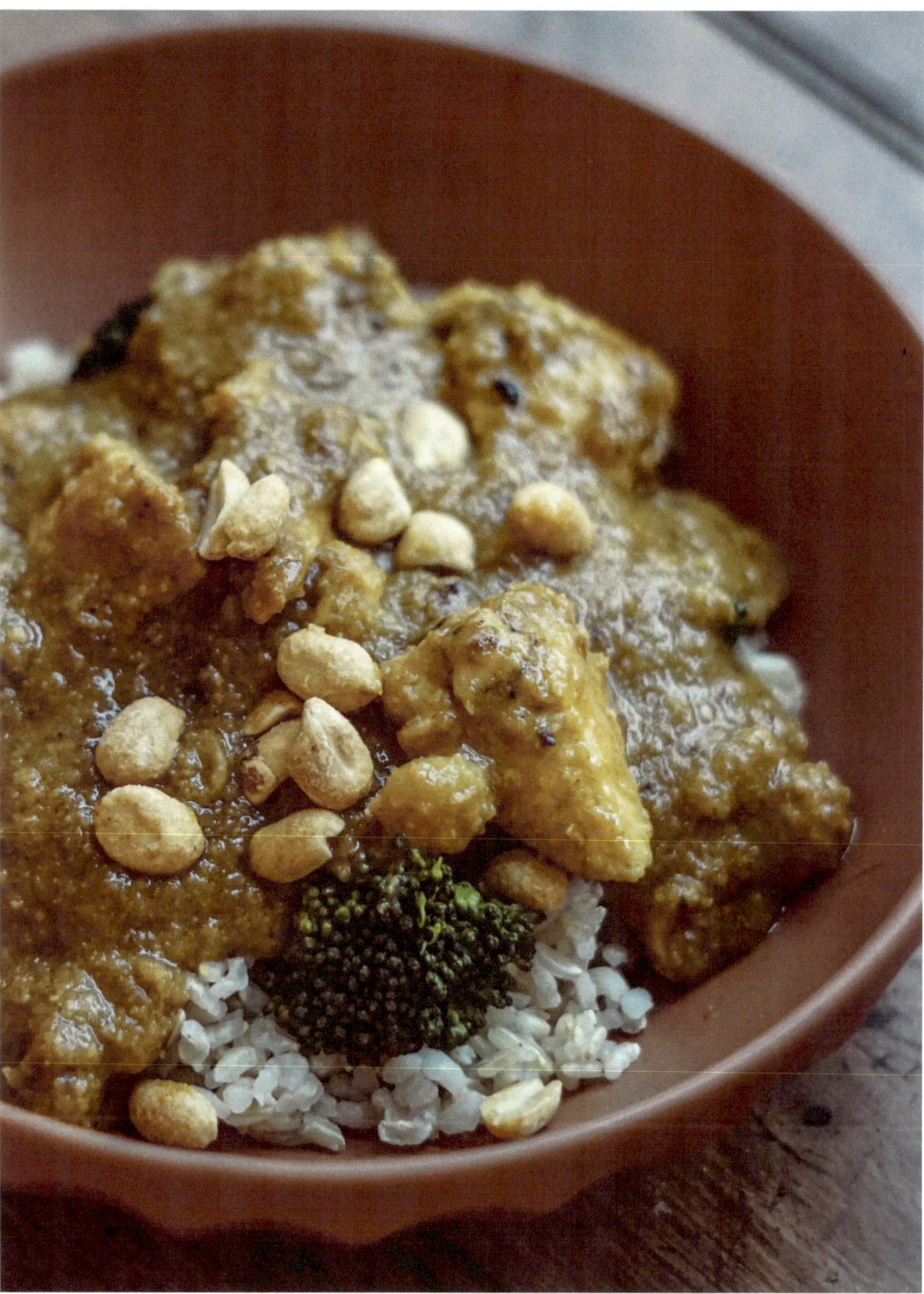

FEELING ADVENTUROUS

PEANUT CURRY

MAKES 4-6 BOWLS

PAIRS WELL WITH:
- CURRY-OSITY (HAD TO DO IT)
- HEAPS OF RICE AND VEGGIES
- PLANT-BASED PEOPLE

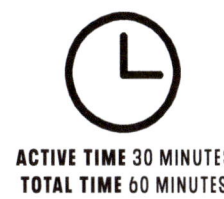

ACTIVE TIME 30 MINUTES
TOTAL TIME 60 MINUTES

SPECIAL EQUIPMENT
Plastic bag or large bowl for marinating
Blender or food processor

INGREDIENTS
SEASONING
1 ½ Tablespoons curry powder
2 teaspoons paprika
2 teaspoons turmeric
2 teaspoons cumin
2 teaspoons coriander
1 ½ teaspoons salt
2 ½ teaspoons sugar
2 pounds chicken thighs, tofu, shrimp or veggies
½ teaspoon chili powder, more if you like it hot

SAUCE
2 Tablespoons soy sauce
2 Tablespoons brown sugar
3 Tablespoons olive oil
3 Thai chilis (adjust to taste)
5 garlic cloves, minced
½ sweet onion
¾ cup chicken broth
1 cup unsalted peanuts
2 Tablespoons peanut butter
1 cup coconut milk - shaken, not stirred

1 Tablespoon soy sauce
2 Tablespoons lime juice
4 lime leaves

SERVE WITH
Rice
Extra peanuts
Lime wedges
Cilantro

INSTRUCTIONS

PREP
Combine all seasoning ingredients in a small bowl, then pour half of that mixture into a plastic bag or bowl large enough to hold your protein.

Prep the protein and add it to the bag or bowl of seasoning. Shake vigorously until evenly coated, then put it in the fridge to marinate (anywhere from one hour to one day).

GET STICKY
A key component of this peanut curry is kecap manis, a sweet, sticky, soy sauce that originates in Indonesia. While the protein marinates, mix two tablespoons of soy sauce and two tablespoons of brown sugar in a small saucepan over medium heat. Simmer the mixture until it starts to get thick and syrupy (about eight minutes), then set aside.

In a separate (large) saucepan, add a tablespoon or two of olive oil, the chilis or chili paste, garlic, and onion. Cook over medium-low heat,t until the onion is translucent.

Add the remaining half of the seasoning and cook until aromatic (another minute or two).

Toss the sticky soy sauce and the chili mixture into your blender and set the saucepans aside. Add the broth and ¾ cup peanuts, then blend until relatively smooth (a few lingering peanut chunks are fine).

CURRY UP
Pour the blended mixture back into the saucepan. Stir in the rest of the peanuts, the peanut butter, coconut milk, additional soy sauce, and lime juice. Mix well.

Grab the lime leaves and squeeze them in your hand to break them up a bit. Add them to the sauce and simmer on medium heat until it starts to thicken (about 15 minutes). It takes time for the lime leaf flavors to really saturate the curry, so we don't recommend rushing this process.

COOK THE PROTEIN
Heat a tablespoon of olive oil in a large pan on medium-high heat, then add your protein to the pan. If using chicken, cook until the internal temp of each "chunk" is 165°F and there's no pink left.

Protein fully cooked? You're ready to serve!

FEELING ADVENTUROUS

TANDOORI-LESS CHICKEN

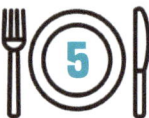

MAKES 5 SERVINGS

PAIRS WELL WITH:
- BORING FOOD BURNOUT
- MASON JAR SALADS
- A BUNCH OF `NAPKINS

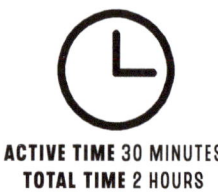

ACTIVE TIME 30 MINUTES
TOTAL TIME 2 HOURS

SPECIAL EQUIPMENT

Baking sheet
Cooling rack
Meat thermometer

INGREDIENTS

8-10 chicken legs or thighs

MARINADE #1
2 Tablespoons lemon juice
2 teaspoons chili powder
2 teaspoons salt

MARINADE #2
1 cup greek yogurt
1 ½ Tablespoons curry powder
1 teaspoon chili powder
1 teaspoon garam masala
3 cloves garlic, minced
½ inch piece of ginger, minced
1 Tablespoon lemon juice
1 Tablespoon olive oil
1 teaspoon salt
¼ teaspoon pepper

SERVE WITH
Leftover marinade #2
Naan or rice
Sauteed veggies

INSTRUCTIONS

First, rinse off the chicken and pat it dry.

In a small bowl mix the lemon juice, chili powder and salt.

Make a few small incisions into each piece of chicken, rub the mixture all over each piece, then place on a baking sheet and toss in the fridge to chill.

While the chicken is marinating (about 20 minutes), mix the greek yogurt, curry powder, chili powder, garam masala, garlic, ginger, lemon juice, olive oil, salt and pepper in a medium-sized bowl.

Remove the chicken from the fridge, coat it with the orange paste you just made, and place it back in the fridge for about 45 minutes.

Preheat the oven to 400°F.

Coat a cooling rack with nonstick spray.

Transfer the chicken onto the cooling rack, then place the rack on a baking sheet.

Bake until the internal temperature of the chicken has reached 165°F (about 30 minutes).

Switch the oven to broil, then cook each side for five minutes. This crisps up the marinade nicely. Be sure to keep an eye on the chicken so it doesn't burn!

Pull the chicken out of the oven, prepare any accompaniments, and enjoy.

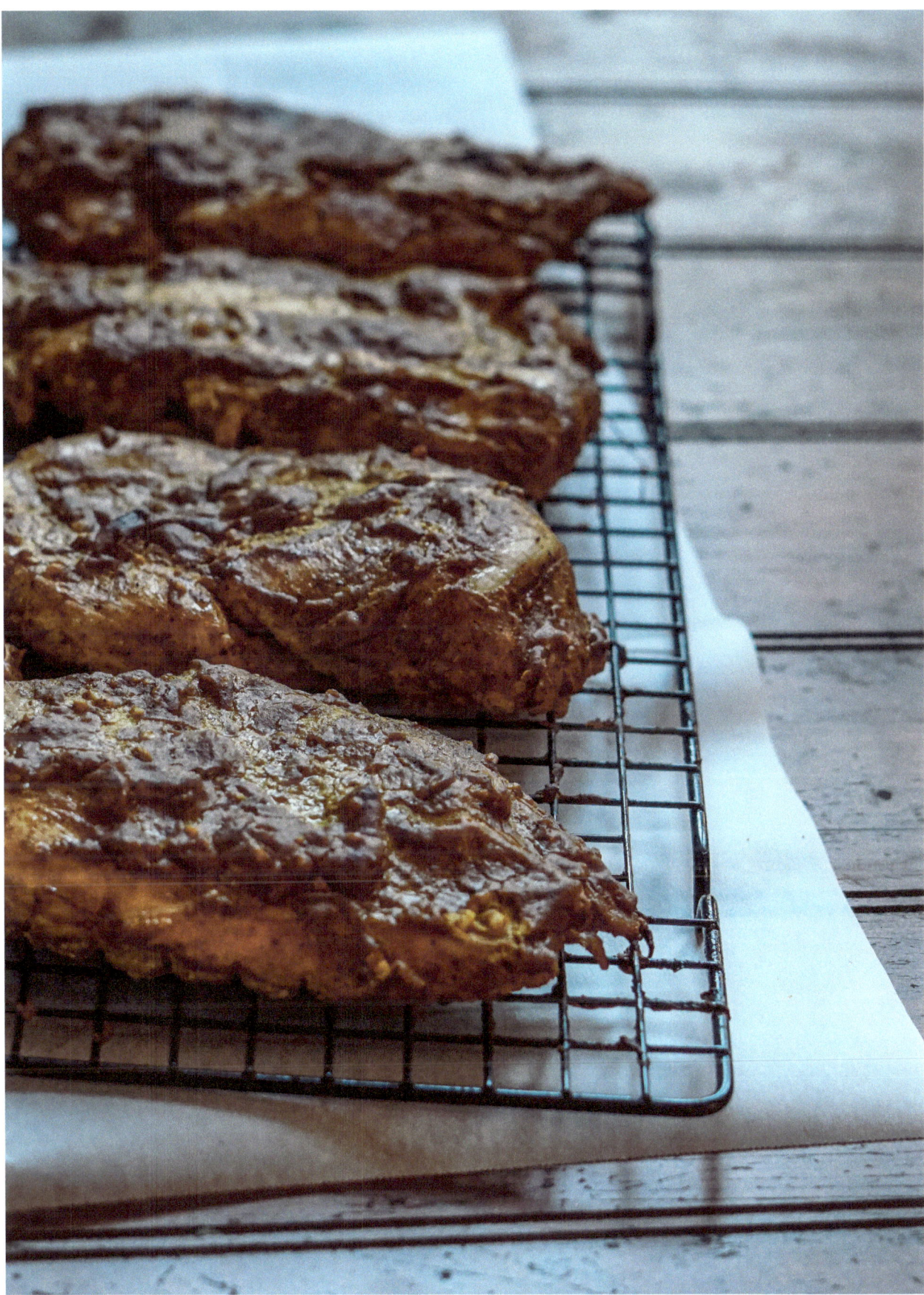

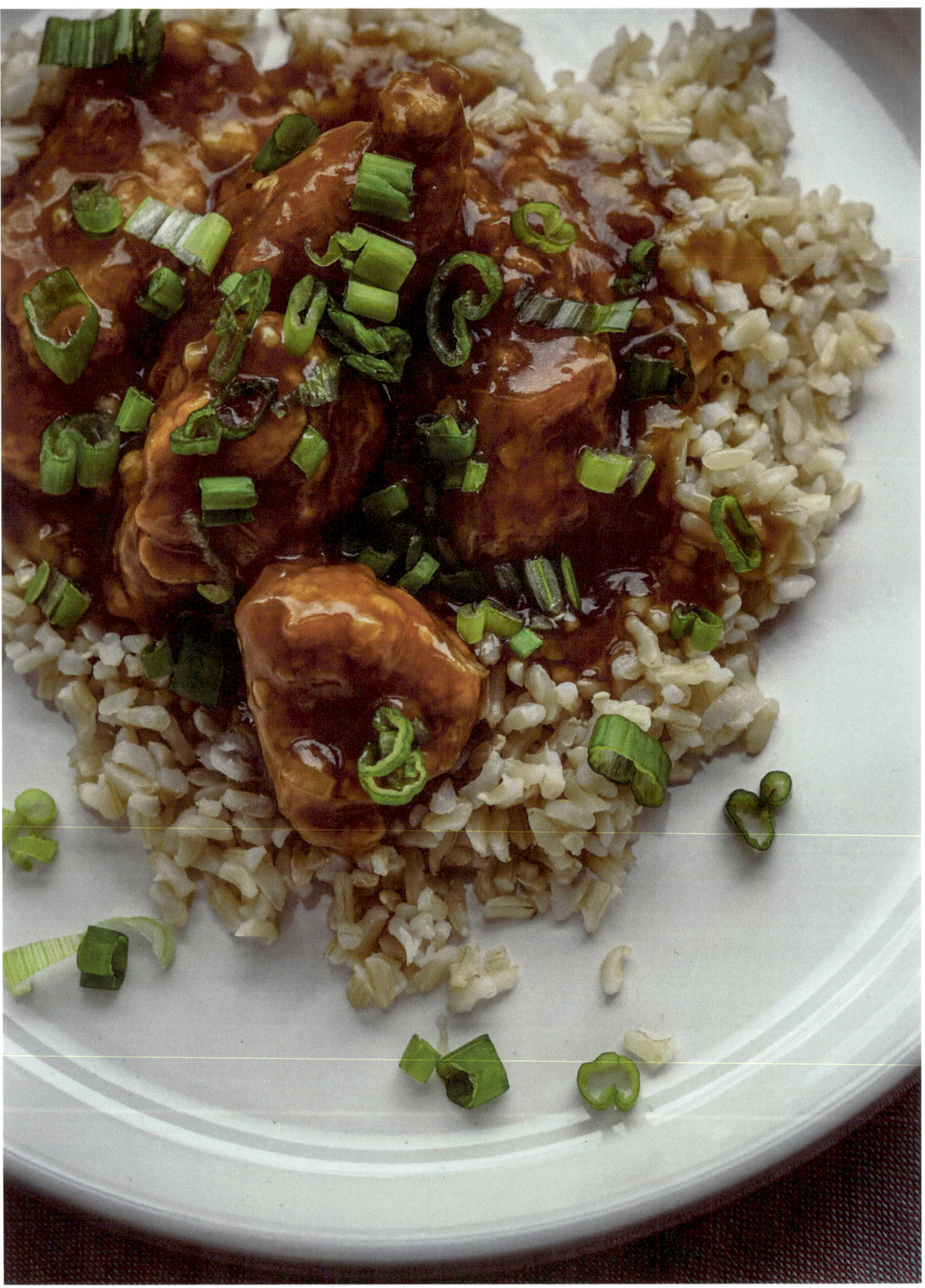

FEELING ADVENTUROUS

SHORT ORDER CHICKEN

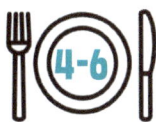

MAKES 4-6 SERVINGS

PAIRS WELL WITH:
- ALL THE SAUCES
- STARTING A NEW TV SERIES
- FRIED CHICKEN SNOBS

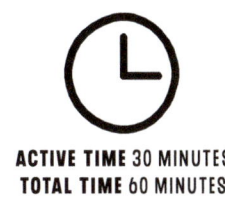

ACTIVE TIME 30 MINUTES
TOTAL TIME 60 MINUTES

SPECIAL EQUIPMENT
Large saucepan or wok
Plastic bag or large bowl for marinating
Meat or candy thermometer

INGREDIENTS

MARINADE
2 egg whites
¼ cup soy sauce
¼ cup shaoxing wine (sub dry sherry if necessary)
¼ cup vodka (very important!)
½ teaspoon baking soda
⅓ cup cornstarch
2 pounds boneless, skinless chicken thighs or breast, cut into chicken nugget-sized chunks

DRY COATING
1 cup flour
1 cup cornstarch
1 teaspoon baking powder
1 teaspoon salt

SAUCE
⅓ cup soy sauce
¼ cup shaoxing wine (sub dry sherry if necessary)
2 Tablespoons cornstarch
¼ cup rice vinegar
⅓ cup chicken stock
½ cup sugar
2 teaspoons toasted sesame oil
1 ½ Tablespoons vegetable oil
1 ½ Tablespoons garlic - minced
1 ½ Tablespoons ginger - minced
1 ½ Tablespoons lemongrass - minced
8 small Chinese chilis (sub ½ teaspoon red pepper flakes)

FINISH
1 ½ quarts vegetable or canola oil

HERE'S THE DEAL
Whether you're craving takeout-style Chinese food or kickass buffalo wings, this may become your new go-to recipe. Keep the marinade, swap the sauce, and voila! Chicken for any occasion.

INSTRUCTIONS

MAKE THE MARINADE
Whisk the egg whites in a large bowl until foamy.
Mix in the soy sauce, wine and vodka, then split the marinade mixture into two bowls.
In one container, add the baking soda and cornstarch. Whisk.
Add the chicken to this half of the marinade and toss thoroughly, then cover and set aside.

DO THE DRY COATING
Mix the flour, cornstarch, baking powder, and salt together. Add the other half of the marinade to the dry ingredients and mix until semi-clumpy. Set this aside.

GET SAUCY
In a small bowl combine the soy sauce, wine, cornstarch, vinegar, chicken stock, sugar and sesame oil until lump free. Set aside.

In a large skillet over medium heat, add the vegetable oil, garlic, ginger, lemongrass and chilis. Cook until soft and fragrant. Stir in the sauce mixture, making sure to get everything out of the bowl. Keep on heat until the sauce boils and starts to thicken, about one to two minutes. Remove it from heat and place it in a bowl to avoid any overcooking.

BRING IT ALL TOGETHER
In a large saucepan or wok, warm the oil to 350°F over medium-high heat, regulating with a meat or candy thermometer. If the oil isn't hot enough, the chicken will be extra greasy. If it's too hot, the chicken won't cook through.

Thoroughly coat each piece of chicken in the dry coating (two to three pieces at a time works best). Using a pair of tongs, gently place each piece of chicken into the oil, one at a time. Cook for four minutes, stirring occasionally to make sure the chicken gets cooked thoroughly. Be careful not to splash hot oil! Use the tongs to remove the chicken and place it on a plate lined with a paper towel.

Toss the chicken and sauce together in a skillet and serve!

FEELING ADVENTUROUS
THAI LAAB SALAD

MAKES 4 CUPS

PAIRS WELL WITH:
- HOT SUMMER DAYS
- EATING ON THE GO
- HEALTH-CONSCIOUS FRIENDS

ACTIVE TIME
30 MINUTES
TOTAL TIME
35 MINUTES

INGREDIENTS
- 1 Tablespoon oil
- 1 pound ground chicken (could swap for any lean protein of choice)
- 1 Tablespoon chili flakes (1 T = medium heat)
- 1 Tablespoon sugar
- 1 Tablespoon fish sauce
- 2 limes, one to juice and one to slice
- 1 shallot, diced
- ½ cup cilantro, chopped
- 4 green onions, chopped
- ⅓ cup mint leaves, chopped

SERVE WITH
Butter lettuce leaves
Rice
Lime wedges

INSTRUCTIONS
- Kick things off by heating the oil in a large pan over medium-high heat.
- Place the chicken (or other protein) in the pan and cook until browned, breaking it up with a spatula while cooking.
- Once the protein is browned, strain off any excess liquid and return it to the pan.
- Stir the chili flakes, sugar, fish sauce, and lime juice into the protein.
- Add the shallot, cilantro, green onion and mint, and mix until everything is well combined.
- Taste and adjust the seasoning as needed (a bit more salt, sugar or fish sauce can help here) to suit your palate, then serve!

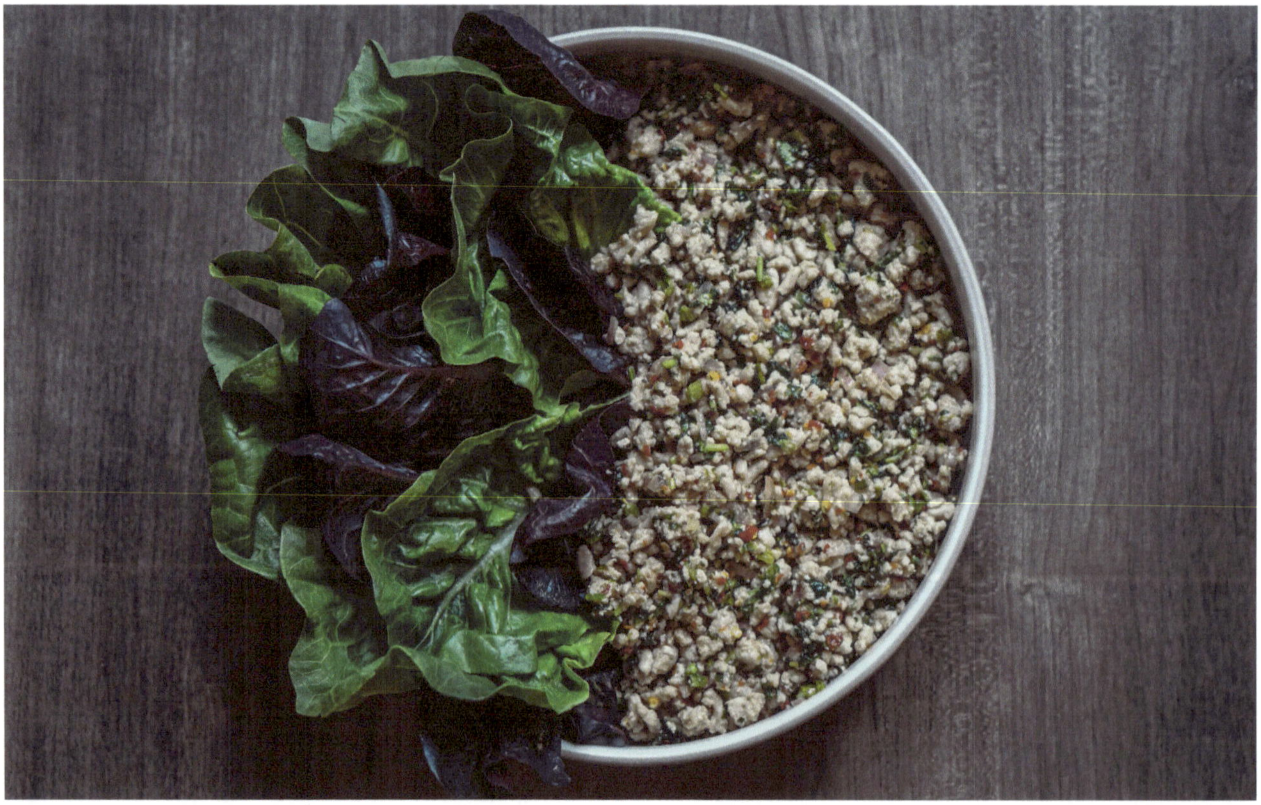

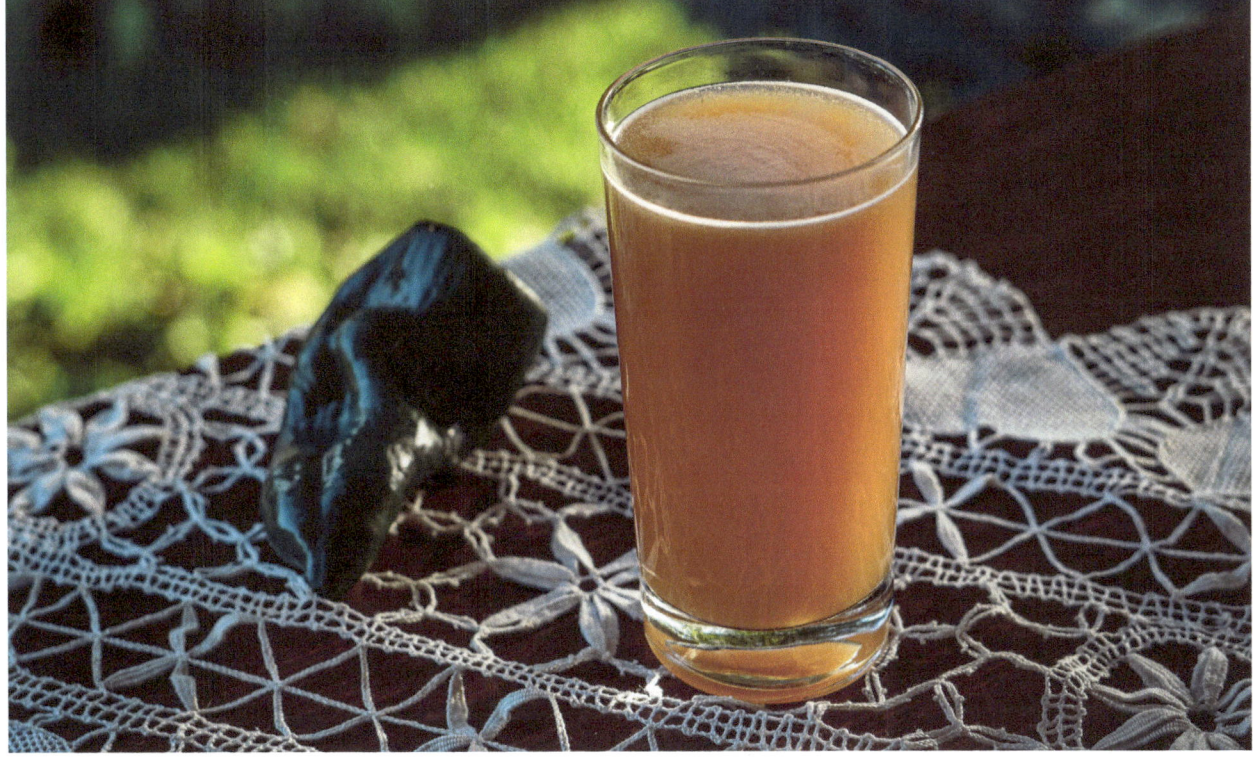

POBLANO PALOMA

MAKES 1 DRINK

PAIRS WELL WITH:
- TROPICAL PRINT
- PRACTICING YOUR SPANISH
- PATIO FURNITURE

SPECIAL EQUIPMENT
Cocktail shaker
Shot glass or liquid measuring device

INGREDIENTS
- ½ grapefruit, juiced
- ½ lime, juiced
- 2 ounces tequila
- ½ teaspoon agave syrup
- ½ poblano pepper, chopped and seeds removed

INSTRUCTIONS
- Combine all ingredients in a cocktail shaker with a handful of ice and shake aggressively.
- Strain into a glass, then pour back into the shaker and strain one more time.
- Garnish however you wish and serve!

LARGER GROUP TIP
Want to stretch your ingredients to make more drinks?
Pour the mixture evenly into each glass and top with soda water.

TOTAL TIME
2 MINUTES

FEELING ADVENTUROUS
WHITE NEGRONI

MAKES 1 DRINK

PAIRS WELL WITH:
- CLASSIC COCKTAIL FATIGUE
- SECOND DATES
- NIGHT CAPS

TOTAL TIME
2 MINUTES

SPECIAL EQUIPMENT
Mixing glass or large cup
Shot glass or liquid measuring device
Rocks glass (recommended)

INGREDIENTS
- 1 ½ ounces gin
- 1 ounce sweet vermouth
- ½ ounce Cocchi Americano
- Lemon peel

INSTRUCTIONS
- Pour the gin, vermouth, and Cocchi Americano into a mixing glass along with a handful of ice.
- Stir until chilled (about 30 seconds).
- Strain the mixture into a rocks glass.
- Use a knife to cut a little peel off of the lemon, then twist it into the glass, releasing some of the juice and oil.
- Run the inside of the peel around the edge of the glass, toss it into the drink (or place it on the rim), and serve!

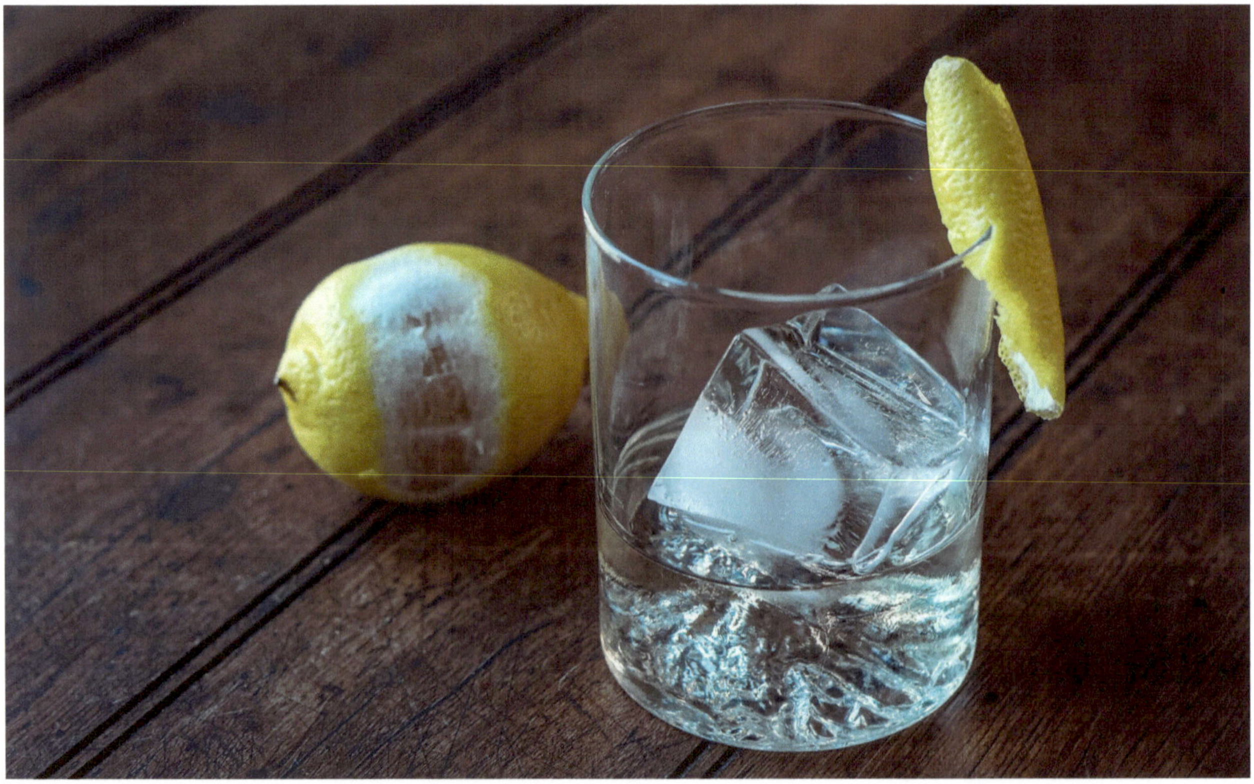

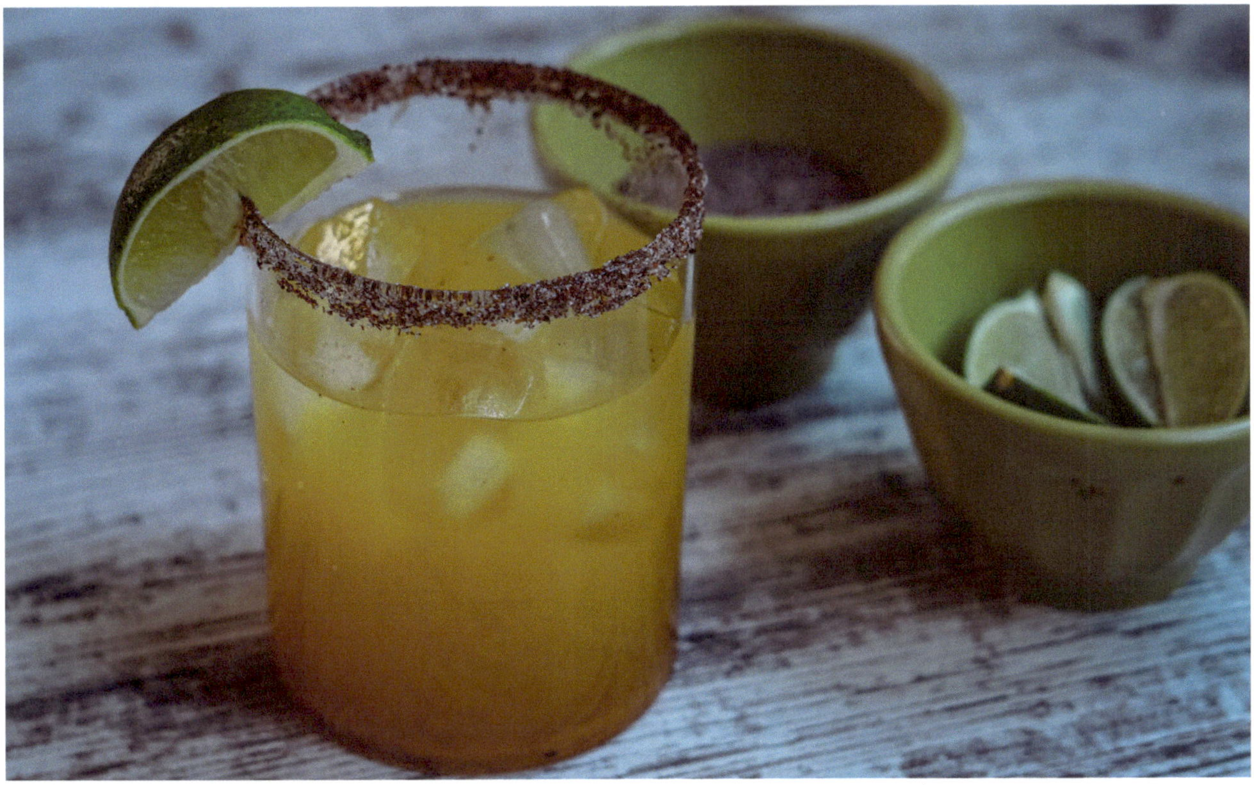

PINEAPPLE TURMERIC MARGARITA

MAKES 1 DRINK

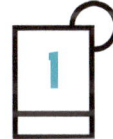

PAIRS WELL WITH:
- MIXING THINGS UP
- HEALTH-CONSCIOUSNESS
- SALSA DIPS AND DANCES

TOTAL TIME
5 MINUTES

SPECIAL EQUIPMENT
Cocktail shaker
Shot glass or liquid measuring device

INGREDIENTS
- 2 ounces tequila
- 2 ounces pineapple juice
- 1 ½ ounces lime juice
- 1 ounce agave syrup
- ½ ounce triple sec
- ¼ teaspoon turmeric, for color

SERVE WITH
- Ice
- Lime wedges
- 1 Tablespoon chili powder
- 1 Tablespoon sugar

INSTRUCTIONS
- Start by mixing together the chili powder and sugar in a bowl or plate, slightly larger than the rim of your glass.
- Use a lime wedge to wet the rim of each glass, then dip into the sugar-chili mixture.
- Combine the tequila, pineapple juice, lime juice, agave syrup, triple sec, and tumeric in a cocktail shaker.
- Top with ice and shake until chilled (about 15 seconds).
- Fill the freshly rimmed glasses with ice.
- Pour, garnish with a lime wedge, and serve!

FEELING

BEAT

FEELING BEAT

CHEAT CODE CHILAQUILES

EASILY FLEXES FOR ANY GROUP SIZE

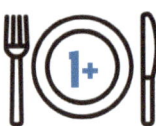

PAIRS WELL WITH:
- HANGOVERS
- STALE TORTILLA CHIPS
- LICKING THE BOWL

TOTAL TIME
10 MINUTES

INGREDIENTS
THE BASICS
- Salsa verde (about 4 ounces per person)
- Tortilla chips
- Eggs

OPTIONAL ADD-ONS
- Canned black beans, drained and rinsed
- Yellow onion, chopped
- Bell pepper, chopped
- Cheese (queso fresco/cotija)
- Cilantro, for garnish

INSTRUCTIONS
Grab a saucepan (the wider the better) and warm the salsa over medium heat.

Add the beans, onion and bell pepper if you like to the saucepan and let simmer for two minutes, then it's time for eggs.

EGG OPTION #1:
Cook the eggs in the simmering salsa (best for 2-4 eggs)

EGG OPTION #2:
Fry the eggs separately (best for large groups)

While you cook the eggs, make a bed of tortilla chips on each bowl or plate for serving.

Spoon a generous amount of salsa goo over the chips and top with as many eggs as you'd like.

Finish with extra peppers or onions, cheese, and cilantro.

Enjoy the dish, then enjoy a nap. You deserve it.

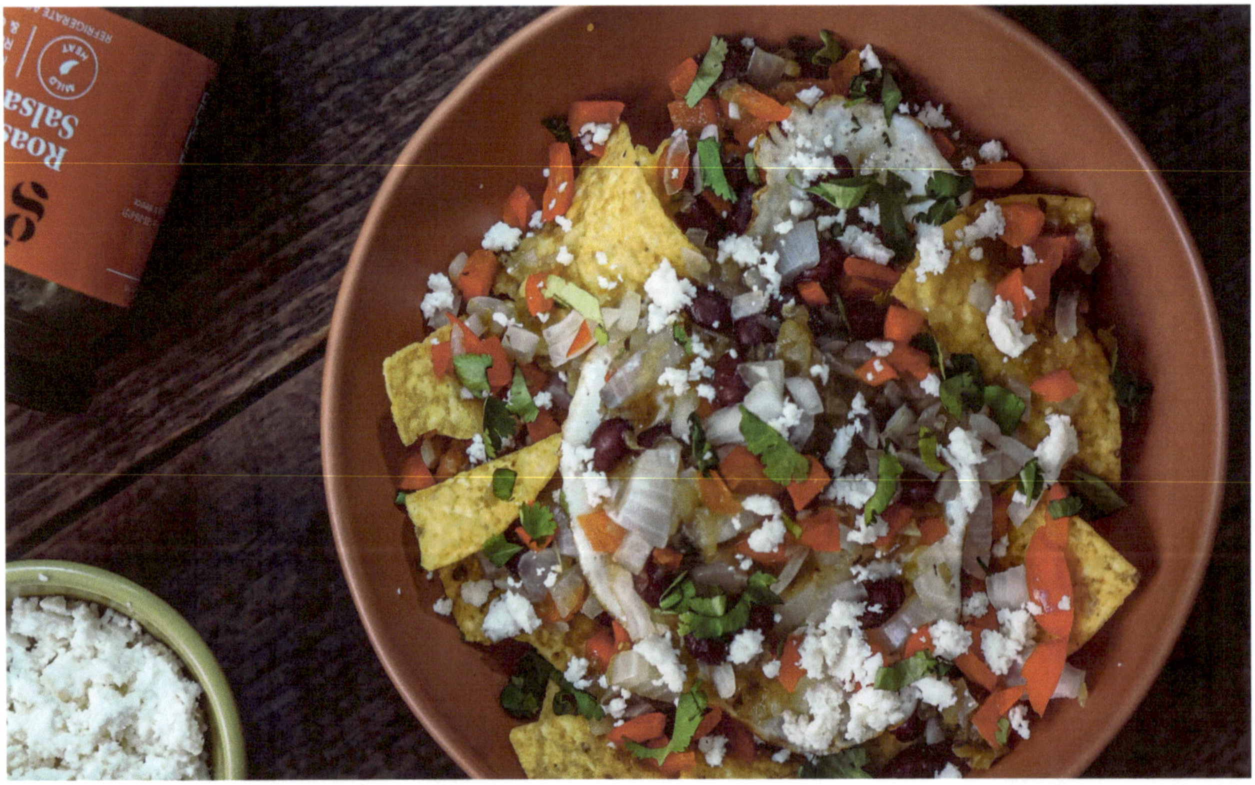

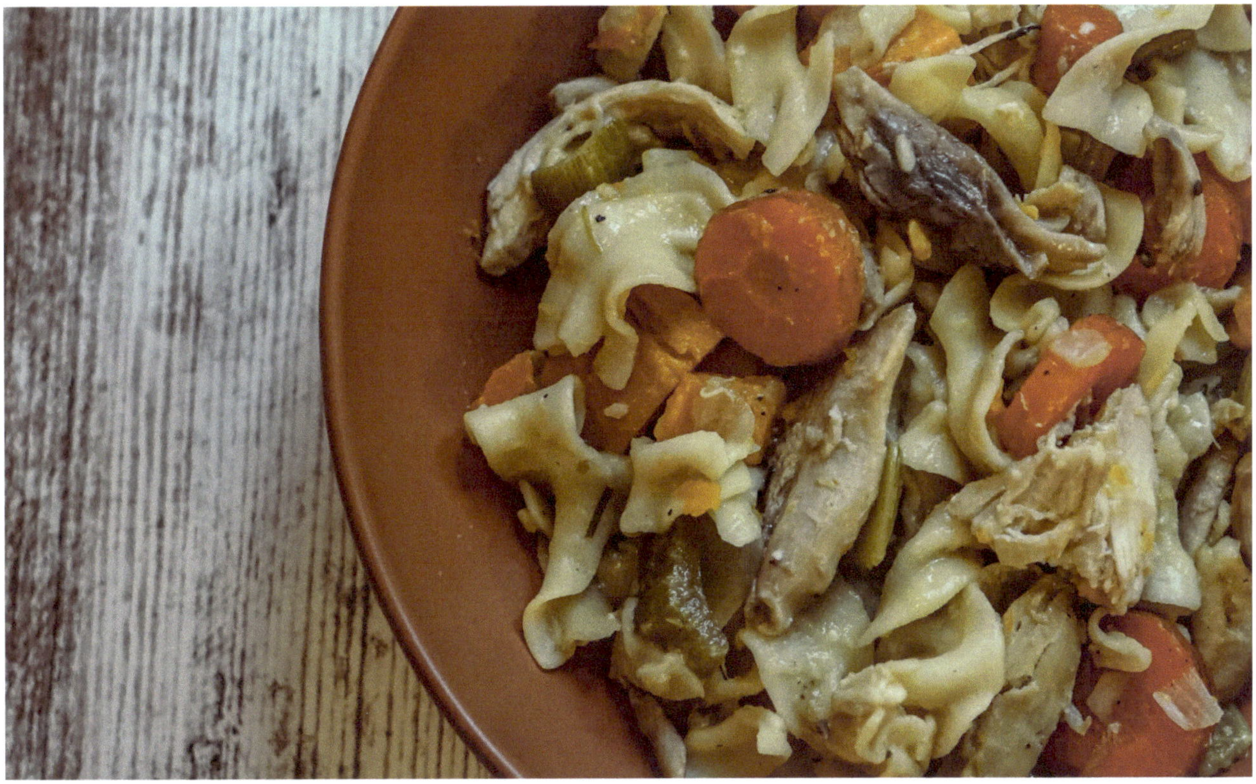

ROTISSERIE CHICKEN NOODLE SOUP

MAKES 4 QUARTS (8-10 BOWLS)

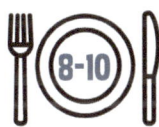

PAIRS WELL WITH:
- COLD & FLU SEASON
- GROCERY SHOPPING WHILE HUNGRY
- SWEATPANTS

ACTIVE TIME
15 MINUTES
TOTAL TIME
30-45 MINUTES

INGREDIENTS
- 2 Tablespoons olive oil
- 1 sweet onion, chopped
- 4 carrots, chopped
- 6 stalks celery, chopped
- 4 cloves garlic, minced
- 1 Tablespoon rosemary
- ½ teaspoon salt and pepper
- 64 ounces chicken broth
- 1 - 12 ounce bag of egg noodles
- 1 sweet potato, peeled and cubed (optional)
- 1 rotisserie chicken, pulled

EASY SWAP
You can substitute three large cooked chicken breasts for the rotisserie chicken if needed.

HERE'S THE DEAL
This soup brings homemade flavor without all the work. Exhausted? Modify as you see fit.

INSTRUCTIONS
- Heat a large stock pot over medium-high heat, then pour in a little olive oil (about two tablespoons).
- Toss in the onion, carrots and celery, and cook until tender (about five minutes).
- Mix in the garlic, rosemary, salt, and pepper and sauté until your kitchen smells noticeably better (about one minute).
- Add the broth, noodles, and sweet potato.
- Bring the pot to a boil, then reduce the heat to medium.
- Simmer until the noodles are cooked, but firm, then add the rotisserie chicken and let it cook until heated throughout (about five minutes).

FEELING BEAT

PEANUTTY PASTA W/BLANCHED KALE

MAKES 4 BOWLS

PAIRS WELL WITH:
- VEGETABLE SKEPTICS
- COLD WINTER NIGHTS
- PEANUT BUTTER FREAKS

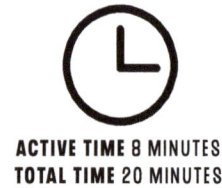

ACTIVE TIME 8 MINUTES
TOTAL TIME 20 MINUTES

SPECIAL EQUIPMENT
Colander/pasta strainer

INGREDIENTS
1 pound pasta
1 large bunch of kale
½ cup peanut butter
½ cup warm water
3 Tablespoons rice vinegar
2 Tablespoons sesame oil
1 Tablespoon ground chili paste or sriracha
1 Tablespoon soy sauce
1 Tablespoon honey
1 Tablespoon lime juice

HERE'S THE DEAL
This is a quick recipe that tastes like it took a long time, and we have yet to meet anyone that doesn't like it.

INSTRUCTIONS
Cook the pasta per the box directions.

While it's cooking, chop or rip the kale into bite-sized pieces, avoiding the bitter stems.

Toss the kale pieces into a colander.

When the pasta is cooked but firm, strain it by pouring the pasta (and water) over the kale.

In a separate bowl, mix the remaining ingredients together until they form a smooth consistency, then it's time to dish!

Portion pasta and kale into bowls and top with a giant scoop of peanut sauce.

Garnish with peanuts, lime slices, and a touch of cilantro if you're feeling crazy.

TWEAK TO YOUR HEART'S CONTENT
Feel free to adjust ingredients to suit your palate. Like spice? Add a little more chili. Sweet tooth? Throw in an extra spoonful of honey.

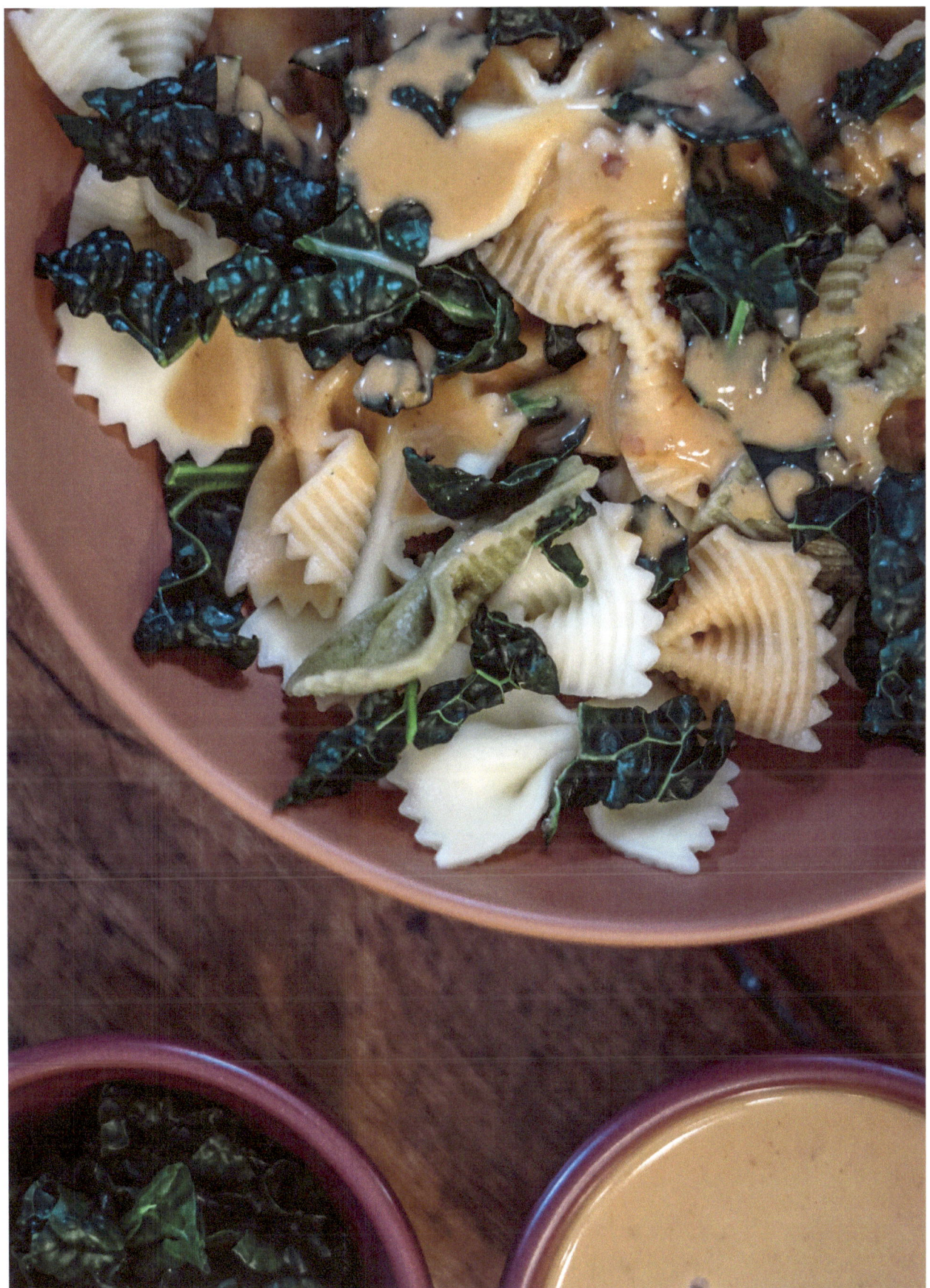

FEELING BEAT

INSTANT ENERGY KALE SALAD

MAKES 2 SALADS

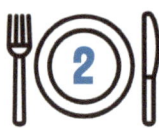

PAIRS WELL WITH:
- IMMUNITY TO CAFFEINE
- LONG WEEKS
- EDIBLE LANDSCAPING

**TOTAL TIME
6 MINUTES**

INGREDIENTS

SALAD
- 1 bunch kale
- 1 teaspoon salt
- 1 sweet apple, chopped
- 2 ounces soft or crumbled goat cheese
- ½ cup granola

DRESSING
- 2 Tablespoons avocado or olive oil
- 1 Tablespoon dijon mustard
- 1 Tablespoon lemon juice
- 1 Tablespoon maple syrup
- Salt and pepper, to taste

HERE'S THE DEAL

Though this recipe does take a small amount of effort, kale packs a nutritional punch that can bring energy back into your day.

INSTRUCTIONS

- Chop or rip the kale off of the bitter stems; aiming for bite-sized pieces.
- Place the kale in a large bowl and massage with a teaspoon of salt until it starts to deepen in color (about one to two minutes), set aside.
- Mix the oil, mustard, lemon juice, syrup, salt, and pepper together.
- Throw this dressing, the chopped apple, goat cheese, and granola into the kale.
- Toss, eat, and enjoy the boost.

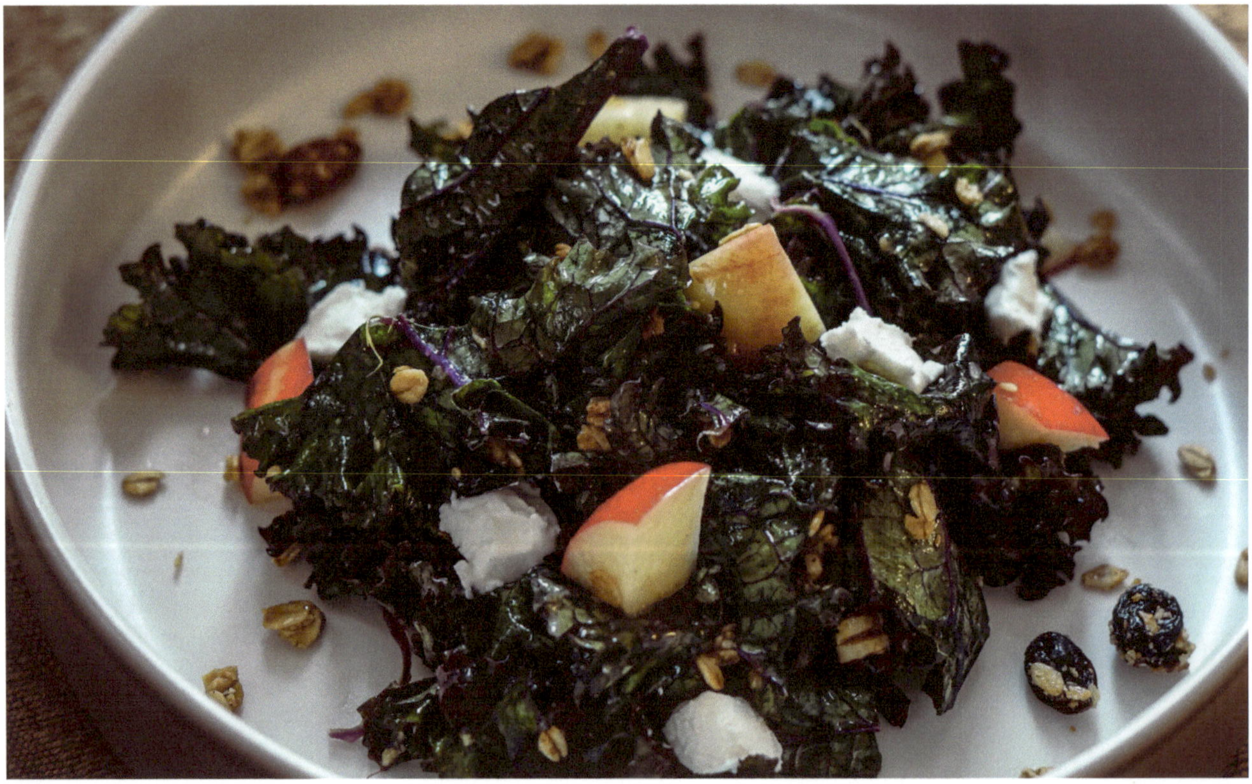

GF

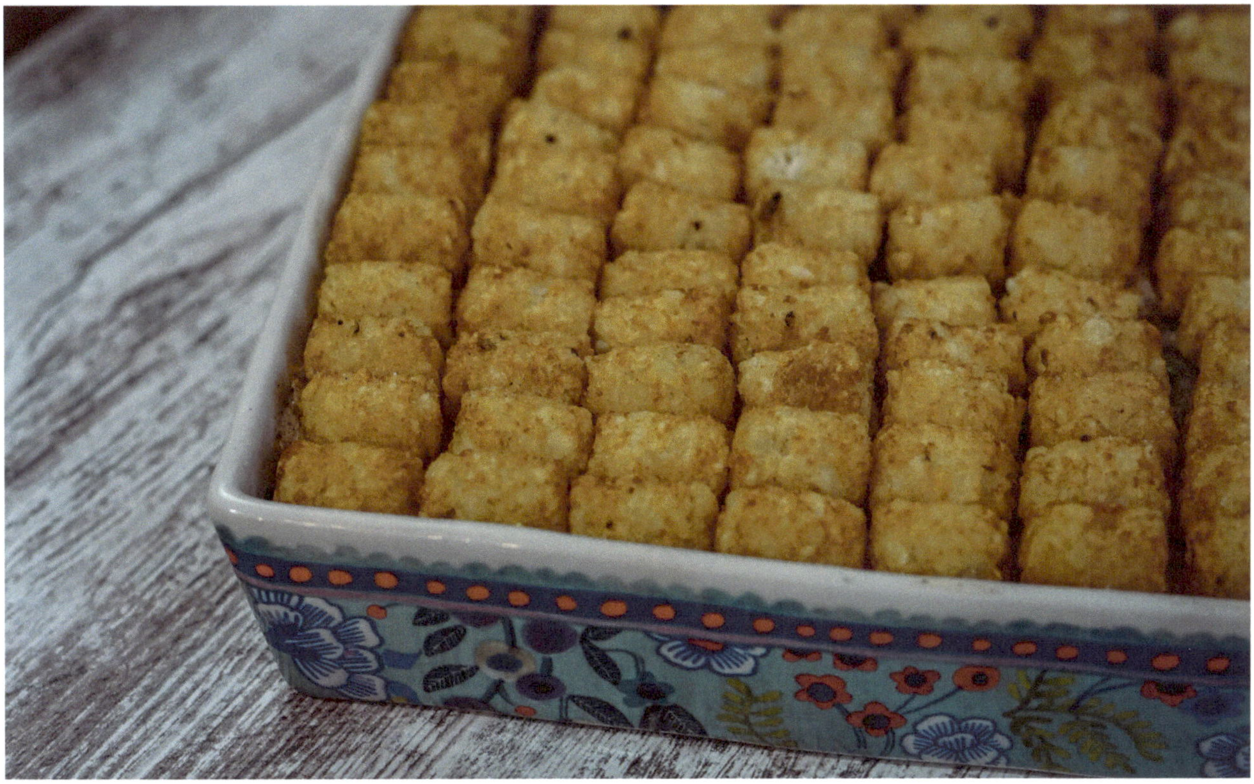

TOTDISH

**MAKES 1 PAN
(6 SERVINGS)**

PAIRS WELL WITH:
- HANGOVERS
- HEAPS OF KETCHUP
- PEOPLE FROM THE MIDWEST

ACTIVE TIME
15 MINUTES
TOTAL TIME
35 MINUTES

SPECIAL EQUIPMENT
10x10 or 9x13 inch baking dish

INGREDIENTS
- 1 pound ground beef
- 1 yellow onion, chopped
- 10.5 ounce can of cream of chicken
- 10.5 ounce can cream of mushroom
- ¾ cup milk
- 16 ounces frozen mixed veggies
- 1 cup cheddar cheese
- 16 ounce bag tater tots

INSTRUCTIONS
- Preheat your oven to 400°F.
- Toss the beef into a fry pan and brown over medium heat.
- While the beef is cooking, chop the onion and add it to the pan.
- Once the meat is fully browned, drain away the grease into a can (not the sink!) and set aside.
- Mix the canned soup and milk in a large bowl, then stir in the veggies, cheese, and beef.
- Pour the mixture into the bottom of the baking dish and evenly place tater tots on top.
- Bake for 30 minutes or until the tots are golden brown and the beef mixture is hot.
- Pull out of the oven, let it cool for a few minutes, and serve!

FEELING BEAT
EASY CARAMEL APPLE DIP

MAKES 1 CUP

PAIRS WELL WITH:
- SPOONS
- POTLUCKS
- TRICKING PEOPLE INTO EATING VEGAN FOOD

TOTAL TIME
5 MINUTES

INGREDIENTS
- ½ cup coconut oil
- ½ cup maple syrup
- ⅓ cup almond butter
- 1 teaspoon vanilla
- Pinch of salt

HERE'S THE DEAL
Maximum yum, minimum effort.

Serve on ginger snaps, apples, fingers... your choice.

INSTRUCTIONS
- Throw all ingredients into a food processor, blender, or for a workout, a bowl.
- Mix well.
- Scoop into a bowl and serve!

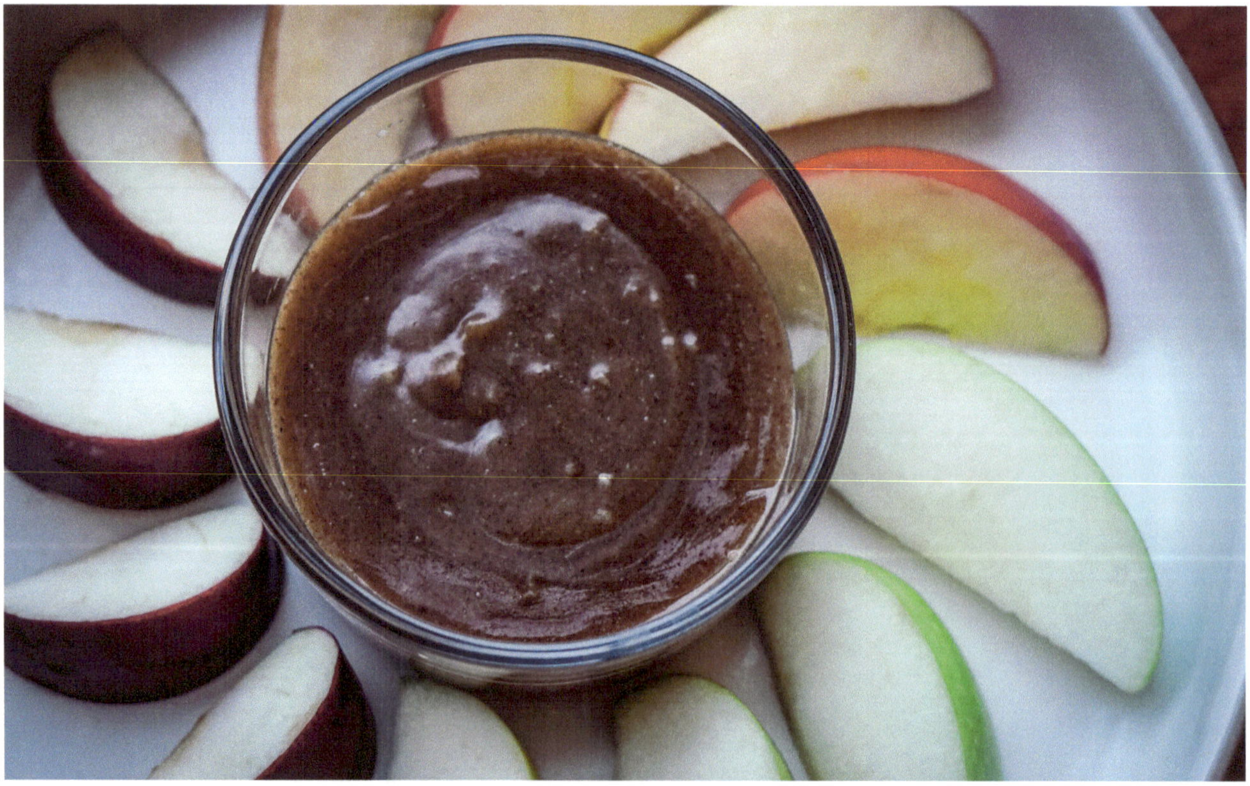

COUNTERTOP TIP
If the dip sits at room temp for awhile, the ingredients may start to separate. Give 'em a quick stir or throw the dip into the fridge and the ingredients will thicken up as they cool.

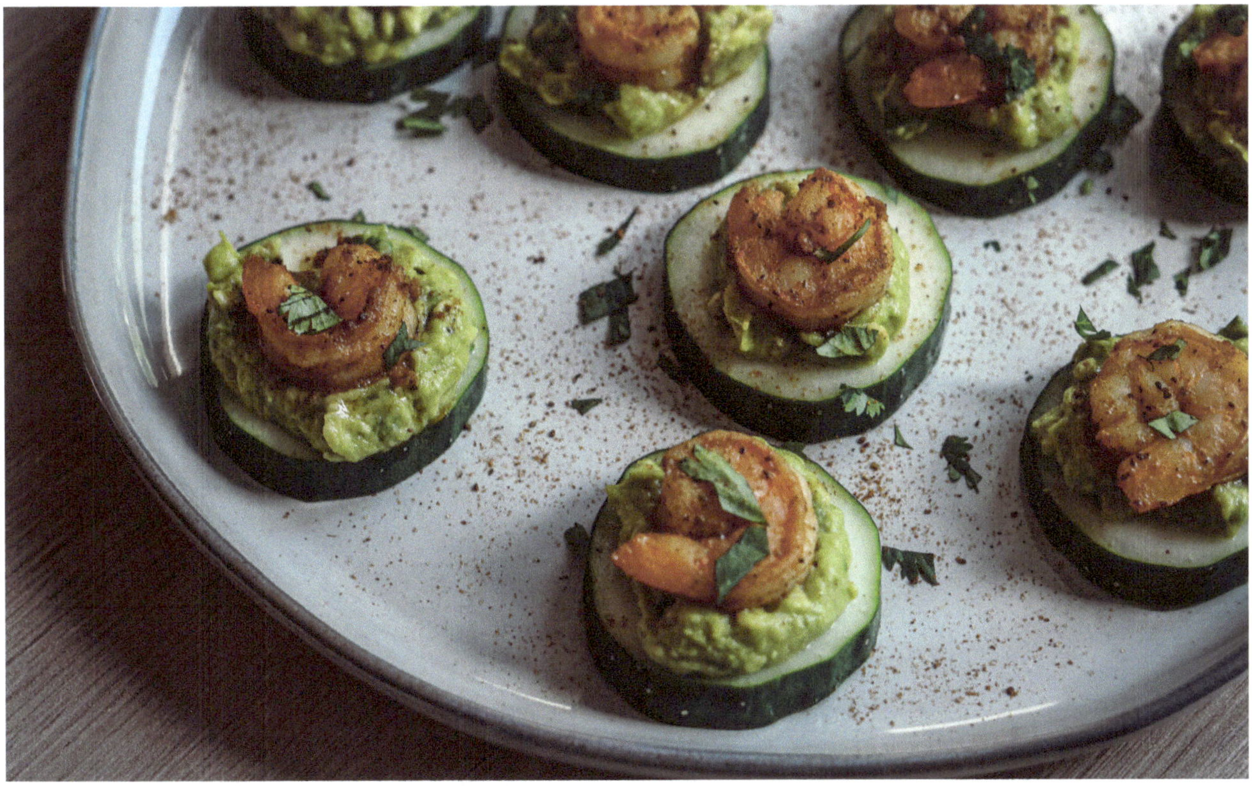

SIMPLE SHRIMP & AVOCADO BITES

MAKES 24 BITES

PAIRS WELL WITH:
- HAPPY HOUR
- HOT DAYS
- DIRTY DISHES

ACTIVE TIME
10 MINUTES
TOTAL TIME
10 MINUTES

INGREDIENTS
- 1 pound raw shrimp, deshelled
- 1 Tablespoon olive oil
- 1 Tablespoon Old Bay seasoning, plus more for garnish
- 1 avocado
- 2 green onions, chopped
- 1 Tablespoon lemon juice
- Salt and pepper to taste
- 2-3 cucumbers, in ¼ inch slices
- 1 Tablespoon cilantro, chopped, for garnish

INSTRUCTIONS
- Toss the shrimp into a bowl with the olive oil and Old Bay seasoning.
- Cook the shrimp over medium heat until it has a little color and is cooked, but not chewy (about two minutes per side).
- Place in a bowl and set aside.
- Cut the avocado in half, then scoop the guts out of its shell and mash it up.
- Mix the green onion and lemon juice into the avocado, then add salt and pepper to taste.
- Lay the slices of cucumber onto a platter or large dish and spoon a small amount of the avocado mash onto each slice.
- Place one shrimp on top of each bite, then garnish with cilantro and a dash of Old Bay and serve!

HOT TIP
If you're using precooked shrimp, you can quickly heat it up in the pan (no more than 30 seconds).

FEELING

BROKE

FEELING BROKE

RENT CONTROL RAMEN $3

MAKES 4-6 BOWLS

PAIRS WELL WITH:
• SAVINGS GOALS
• SOY EGGS (NEXT PAGE)
• SLURPING NOISES

TOTAL TIME
5 MINUTES

INGREDIENTS
- 4 ramen packages
- ⅓ cup tahini
- 1 Tablespoon maple syrup
- 3 green onions, chopped

INSTRUCTIONS
- Cook the ramen noodles according to package instructions, then drain about half the water from the pot.
- Add the ramen seasoning packets, tahini, and maple syrup.
- Stir until the broth forms a creamy consistency.
- Toss in the green onion, remove from heat, and serve!

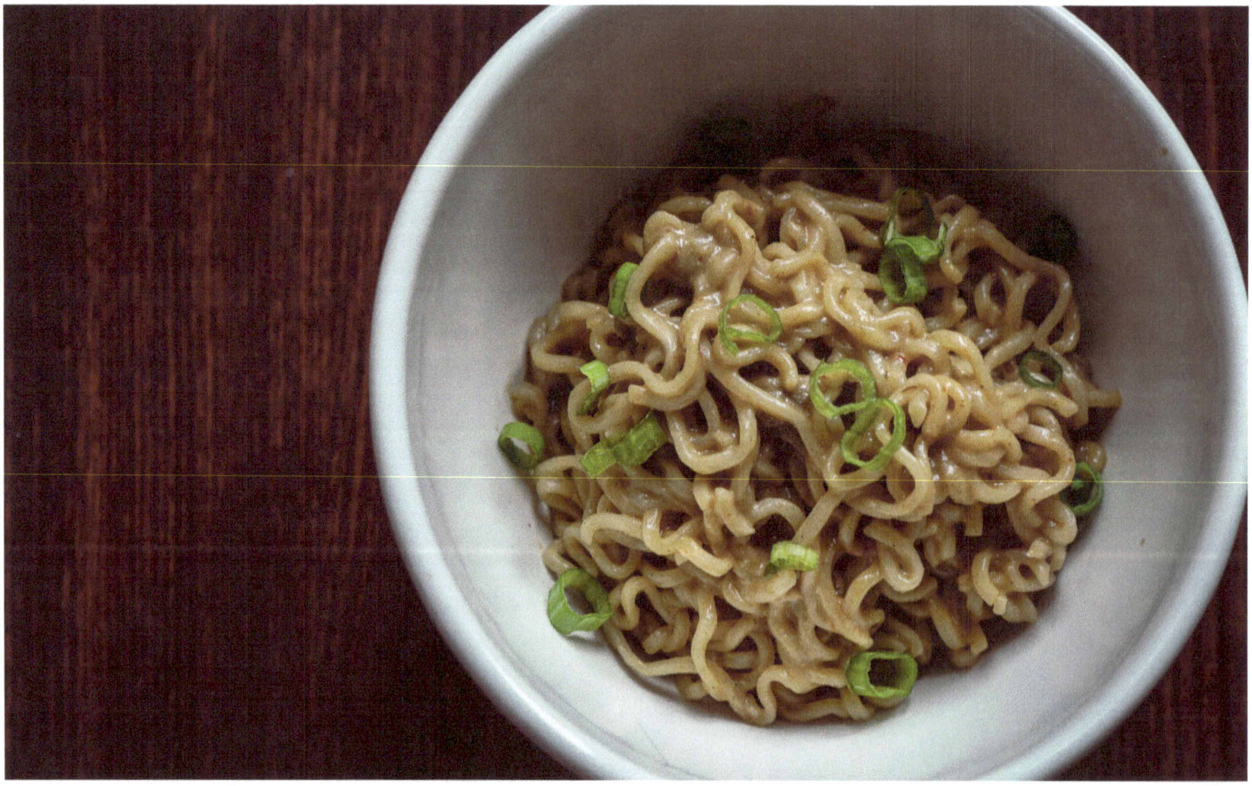

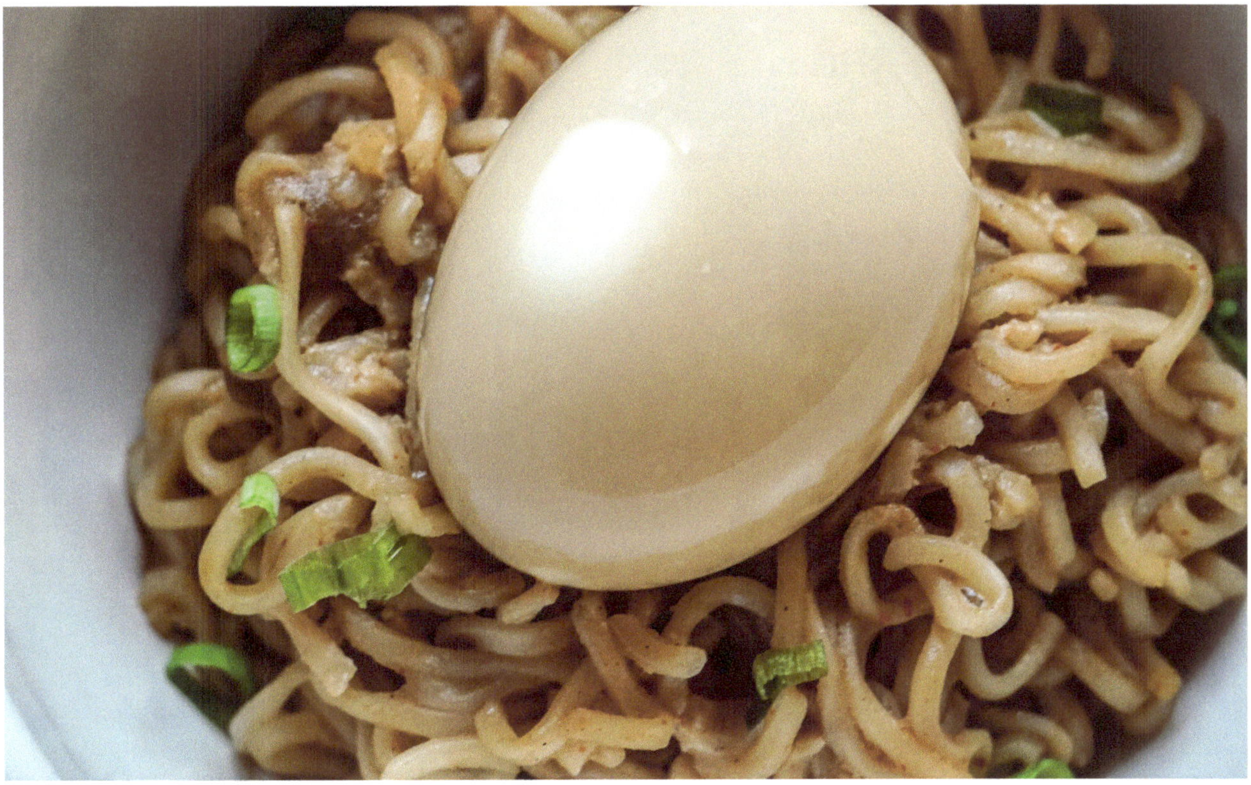

SOY CHEAP EGGS $0.85

MAKES 6
MARINATED EGGS

PAIRS WELL WITH:
- OVERDRAFT FEES
- FANCY INSTANT RAMEN
- CHAMPAGNE TASTES + BEER BUDGETS

ACTIVE TIME
8 MINUTES
TOTAL TIME
1 HOUR 8 MINUTES

HERE'S THE DEAL
Use this as your go-to recipe for perfectly boiled eggs (stop when you hit "ice water") or continue for flavor-rich soy eggs that add something special to a bowl of instant ramen.

INGREDIENTS
- 6 eggs
- 1 Tablespoon powdered sugar
- 3 Tablespoons apple cider vinegar
- ⅓ cup soy sauce

A SWEET TIP
If you don't have powdered sugar, you can toss some normal sugar into a blender.

INSTRUCTIONS
- Gently place the eggs into a medium-sized pot, then fill the pot with water until the eggs are covered.
- Boil for eight to 10 minutes.
- While the eggs are boiling, mix together the other ingredients in a bowl or tupperware container (ideally with a lid) and fill a separate bowl with ice water.
- Transfer the eggs from the pot to the ice water.
- Once the eggs are cool enough to handle, peel them!
- Start by cracking the shell on a flat surface, roll to loosen the shell, and peel away.
- Place the peeled eggs in the marinade for at least an hour, flipping them every 30 minutes to get that saturated soy goodness on all sides.
- Add the eggs to a fancy instant ramen, chop them and throw them in a salad, or eat them right out of the container. Enjoy!

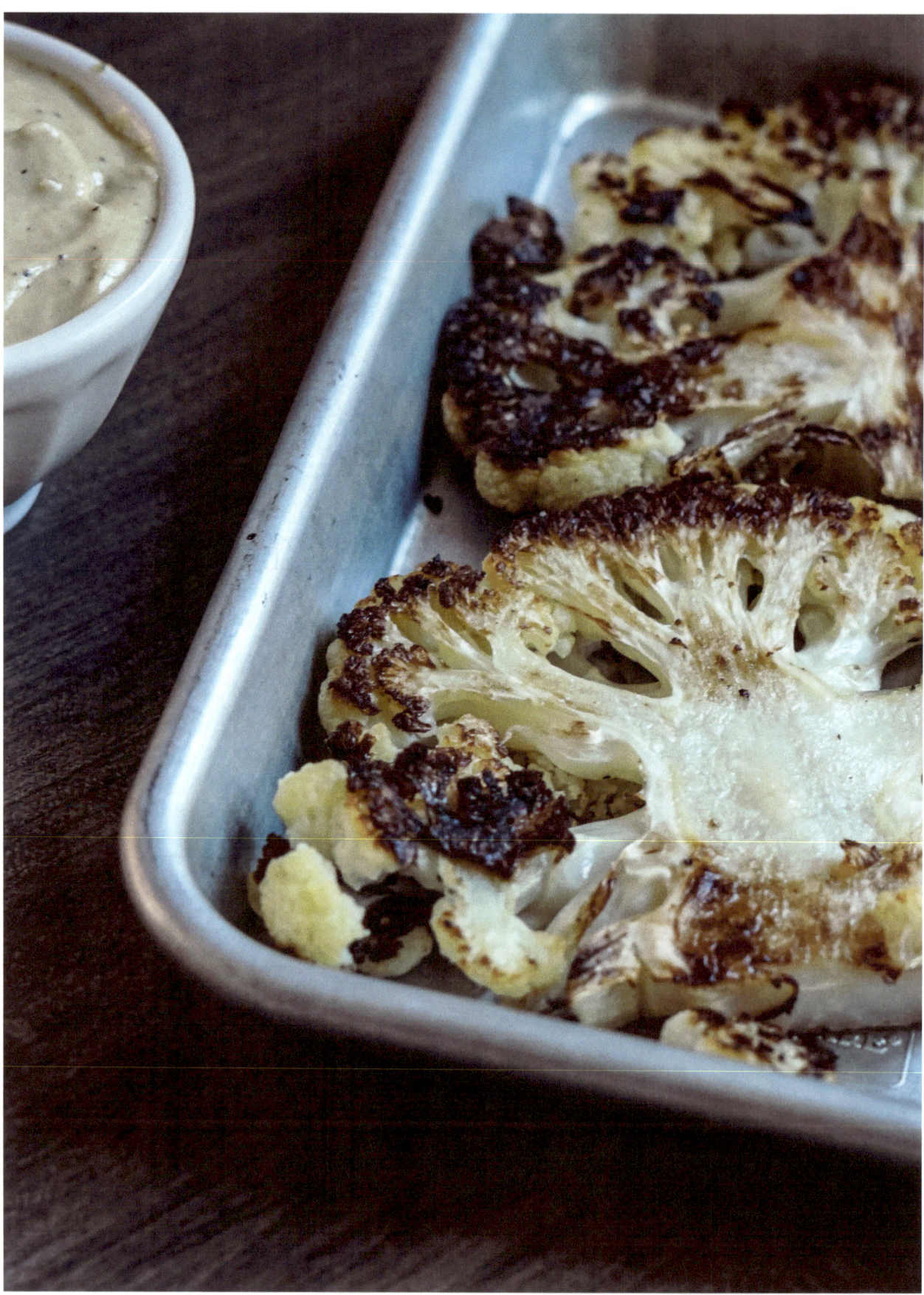

FEELING BROKE

CASH-STRAPPED CAULIFLOWER STEAKS $3

MAKES 2 STEAKS + A BUNCH OF CRUMBLES

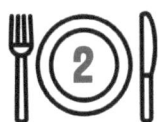

PAIRS WELL WITH:
- VEGETARIANS
- FOODIES
- BEGINNERS

ACTIVE TIME 10 MINUTES
TOTAL TIME 40 MINUTES

INGREDIENTS

CAULIFLOWER STEAKS

1 cauliflower head
2 Tablespoons olive oil
Salt to taste

DIJON AIOLI

¼ cup mayo
2 Tablespoons olive oil
2 Tablespoons dijon mustard
1 teaspoon garlic
Salt and pepper to taste

HERE'S THE DEAL

If you panicked at "aioli," stick with us. This recipe is easy and SO good.

INSTRUCTIONS

Preheat the oven to 450°F. Line a baking sheet with aluminum foil, then coat the foil with cooking spray.

Grab the cauliflower, then use a sharp knife to cut away the leafy parts from the stems.

Cut the head down the middle, right through the core, then cut each half in half again, creating four cauliflower "steaks." If the two smaller steaks start to crumble and turn into florets, no worries - they will still be delicious.

Place each "steak" (and any leftover crumblies) on the baking sheet and drizzle with olive oil. Sprinkle with salt and pepper, flip, and repeat.

Place the baking sheet on the middle rack of the oven and bake until the cauliflower is golden brown (about 25 minutes), flipping once in the middle.

While the steaks are in the oven, mix the mayo, olive oil, dijon mustard, garlic, salt, and pepper in a small bowl to create the aioli.

Once the cauliflower is golden brown, pull it out of the oven and let it rest for about five minutes.

Drizzle the aioli over the cauliflower and you're ready to eat!

FEELING BROKE

CHOCOLATE PB DROP COOKIES $3

MAKES 12 DELICIOUS BLOBS

PAIRS WELL WITH:
- FISCAL RESPONSIBILITY
- ALL THE MILKS
- CHOCOLATE CRAVINGS

TOTAL TIME
15 MINUTES

SPECIAL EQUIPMENT
Wax paper

INGREDIENTS
- 1 cup sugar
- ¼ cup milk
- ¼ cup butter
- 1 ½ Tablespoons cocoa powder
- ½ teaspoon salt
- ½ teaspoon vanilla
- 1 cup peanut butter
- 1 ½ cups quick oats

INSTRUCTIONS
- Combine the sugar, milk, butter, and cocoa in a pot over medium heat.
- While stirring, bring the mixture to a full boil for 90 seconds, add the salt and vanilla, then reduce the heat to medium-low.
- Stir in the peanut butter and mix until smooth, then remove from heat and stir in the oats.
- Use a spoon to "drop" scoops of the mixture onto a sheet of wax paper.
- Let the cookies cool for a few minutes while you enjoy the smells, then enjoy!

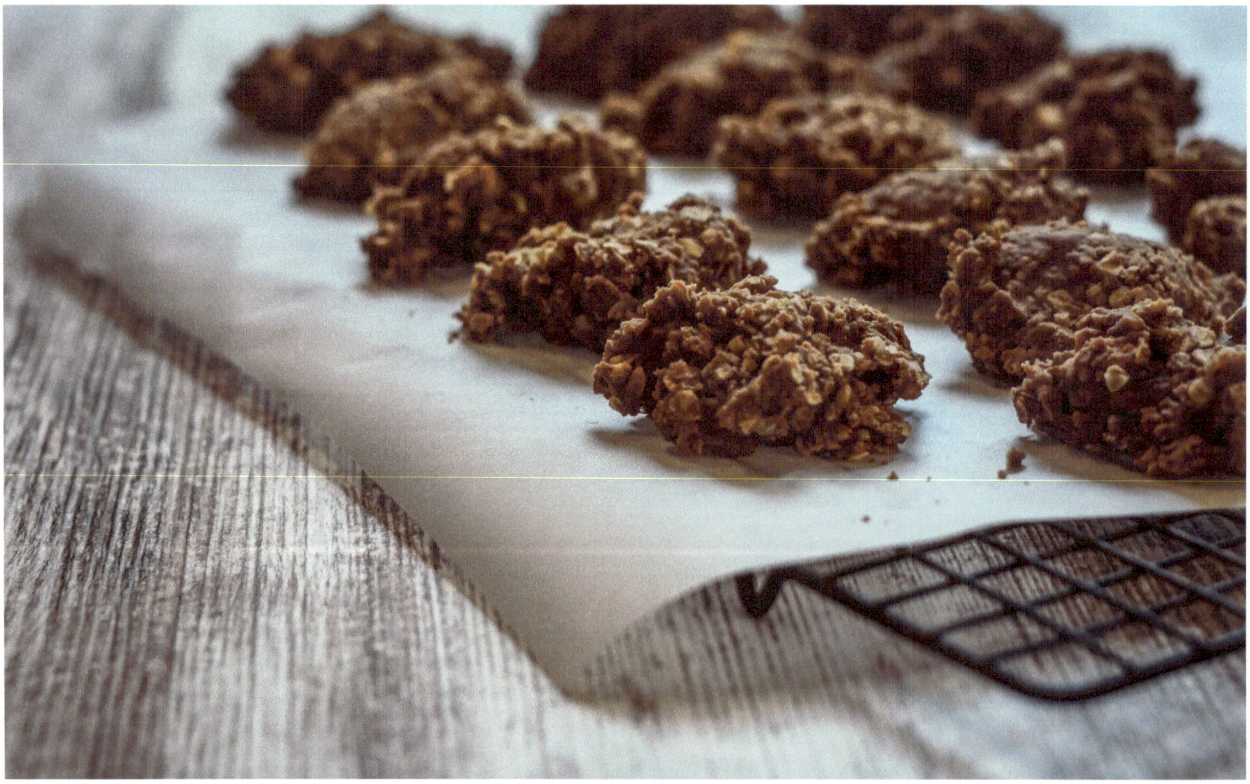

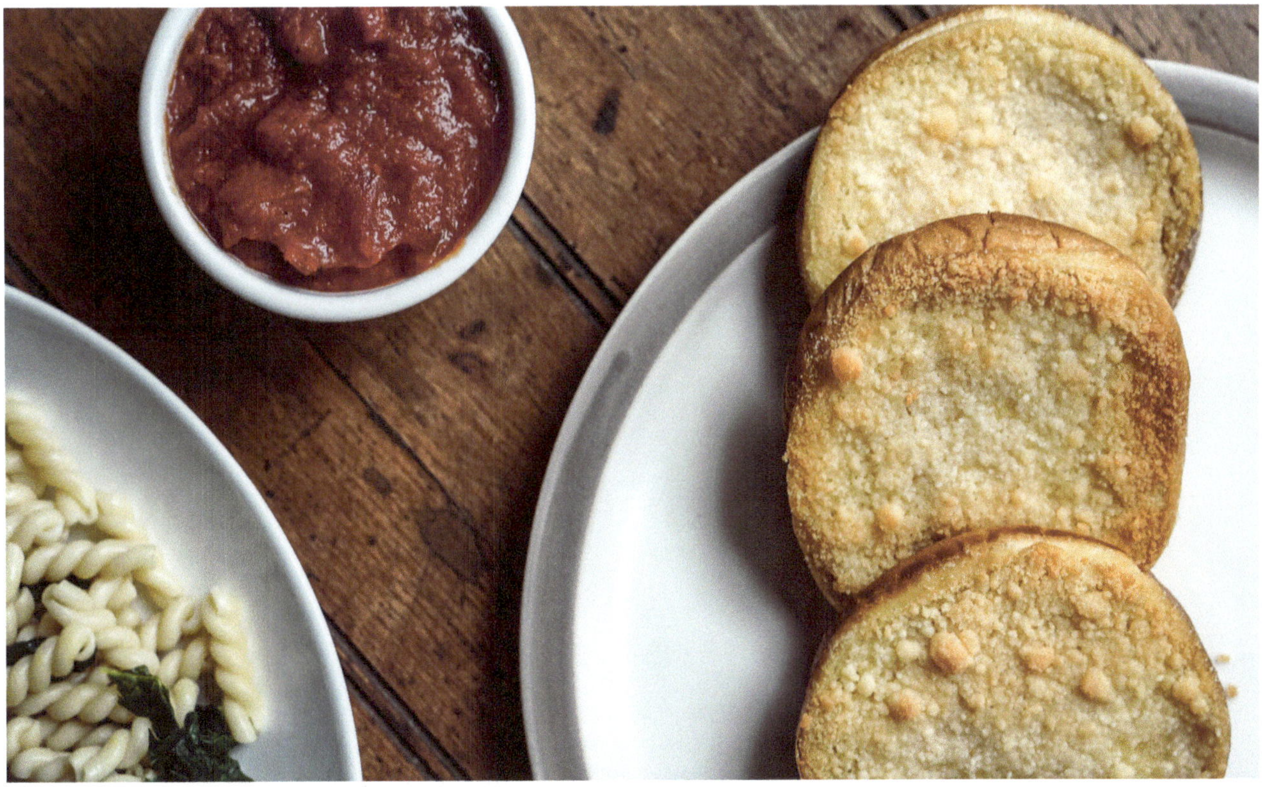

GRANDMA NIXA'S BUNS $2.35

MAKES A BUNLOAD OF CHEESY TOAST

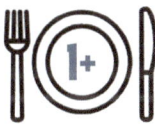

PAIRS WELL WITH:
- OVERDUE RENT
- STALE BREAD
- SAUCE. RED SAUCE.

TOTAL TIME
10 MINUTES

INGREDIENTS
- Butter, room temperature
- Hamburger buns (as many as you can eat)
- Parmesan cheese, grated

INSTRUCTIONS
- Call your Grandma and say hi while you preheat the oven to 350°F.
- Spread a thin layer of butter on each bun, then sprinkle with a generous amount of parmesan.
- Place eat piece on a baking sheet (parmesan-side-up) and cook until golden brown (about five minutes).
- Remove from the oven and serve with marinara sauce.

FEELING BROKE

BUDGET BRUSCHETTA $4.25

**MAKES 1 LOAF
(ABOUT 12 SLICES)**

PAIRS WELL WITH:
- COMMUNITY GARDENS
- NEWLYWEDS
- BOUGIE FRIENDS

ACTIVE TIME
10 MINUTES
TOTAL TIME
15 MINUTES

SPECIAL EQUIPMENT
Cheese grater
Baking sheet

INGREDIENTS
- 3 large tomatoes
- 1 large loaf of bread - baguette or ciabatta work well
- Olive oil
- Salt
- Fresh basil

INSTRUCTIONS
- Preheat the oven to 350°F.
- Find the largest option on your cheese grater, then grab each tomato and "grate" it into a bowl. This may seem odd, but trust us, this technique has a yummy result. Be careful not to grate your fingers!
- Slice the bread into mouth-sized pieces (about ½ inch), then drizzle with olive oil.
- Place the bread onto a baking sheet and toast in the oven until it's warm and slightly crisp (about five minutes).
- Once the bread is out of the oven, spoon some tomato onto each piece and drizzle generously with olive oil.
- Sprinkle with salt, top with a basil leaf, and go!

GRATE JOB
No cheese grater? Cut a tomato in half, then rub it on each slice of the freshly toasted bread.

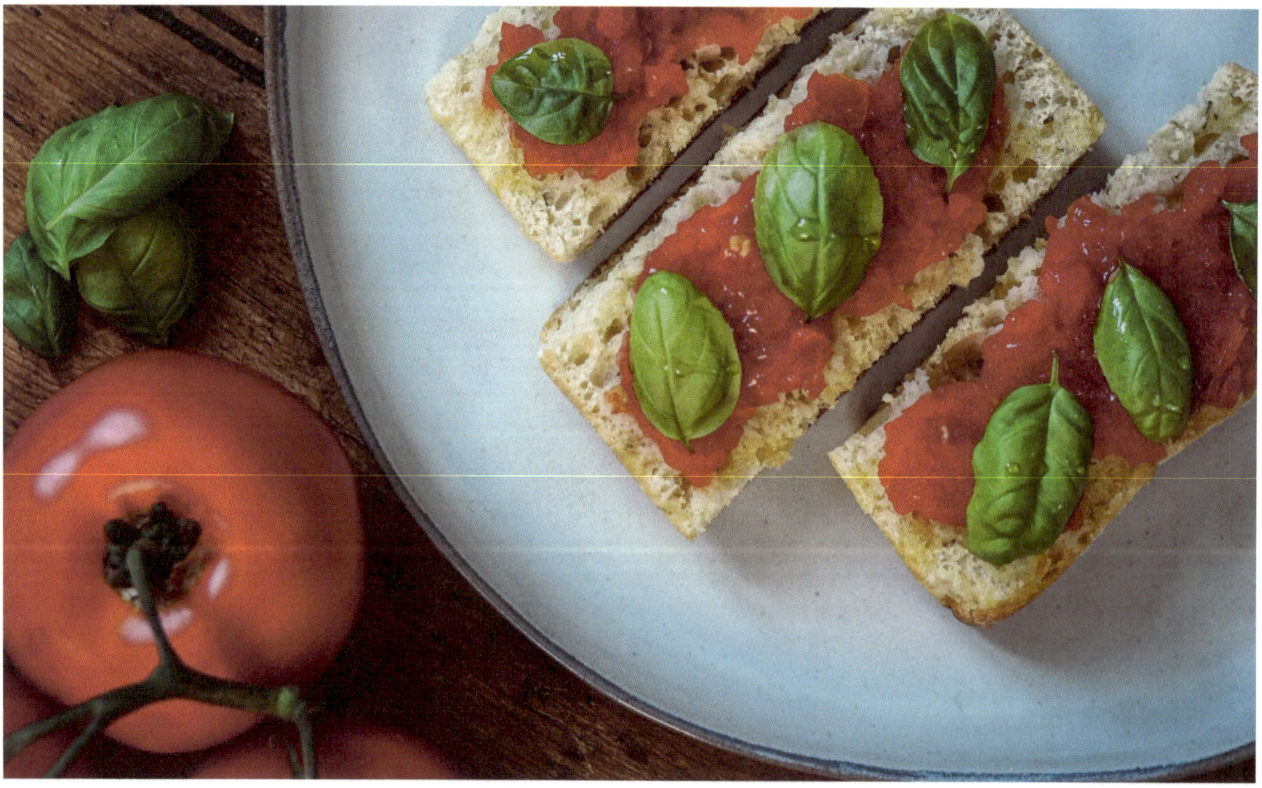

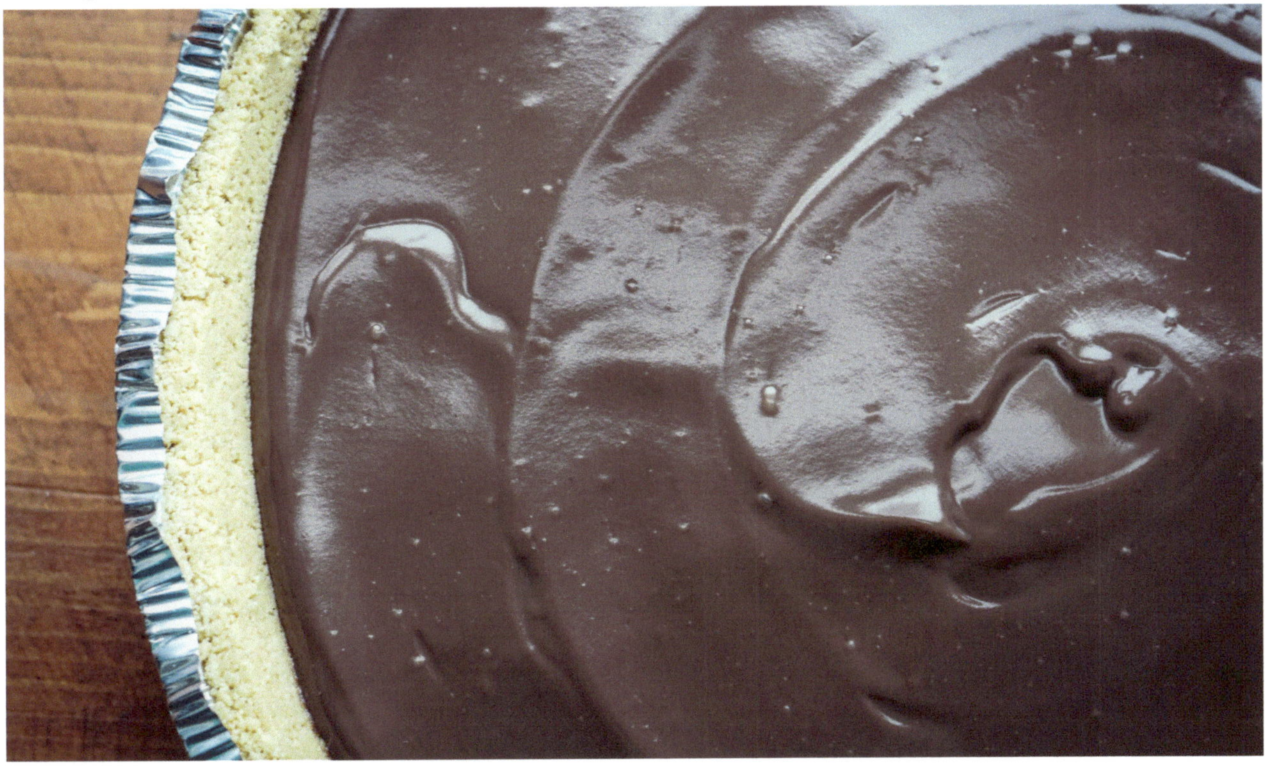

PUDDIN' MYSELF THROUGH COLLEGE PIE $2.95

MAKES 1 PIE

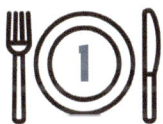

PAIRS WELL WITH:
- LATE DENTAL PROCEDURES
- ROOMMATES
- CHOCOLATE CRAVINGS

TOTAL TIME
5 MINUTES

INGREDIENTS
- 1 box instant chocolate pudding
- 2 cups milk (per pudding instructions)
- 1 store-bought graham cracker crust
- Whipped cream (optional)

INSTRUCTIONS
- Pour the pudding mix into a large bowl, then whisk in the milk. Continue whisking for two minutes or until the pudding starts to thicken. If these aren't the directions for your box of pudding, follow those. We don't know everything.
- Scoop the pudding into graham cracker crust and top with whipped cream (if you like).
- We recommend refrigerating for about one hour to ensure the pudding gets nice and firm, but if you're too hungry to wait, grab a spoon. We won't judge.

FEELING BROKE

PIZZA (DOUGH) $1.75+TOPPINGS

MAKES 3 CRUSTS

PAIRS WELL WITH:
- LEFTOVERS
- LARGE GROUPS
- LITTLE HELPERS

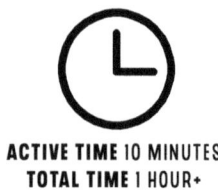

ACTIVE TIME 10 MINUTES
TOTAL TIME 1 HOUR+

HERE'S THE DEAL

This recipe covers the most essential part of a good pizza - the crust! Once you've made the dough, you can load it up with your favorite ingredients or store it for future pizza making.

SPECIAL EQUIPMENT

Pizza stone (optional but useful for crispy crust)

INGREDIENTS

4 ½ cups flour (use bread flour for thicker crust, all-purpose flour for thinner crust)
2 teaspoons salt
1 teaspoon instant yeast
¼ cup olive oil
1 ¾ cups cold water

INSTRUCTIONS

IF MIXING BY HAND...

- In a large bowl, whisk together the flour, salt and yeast.
- Stir in the oil and water until well combined.
- Knead the dough, until it's nice and smooth (about five minutes).
- If the dough is still sticky after five minutes, add a small amount of flour, then knead until it's no longer sticky (about 30 seconds).

IF USING A STAND MIXER...

- Mix the flour, salt, and yeast on low (unless you want to decorate your kitchen with flour).
- Add in the oil and water and mix with a paddle attachment until they are well combined into the dough (about 30 seconds).
- Switch to the dough hook, then knead at a medium speed for five minutes.
- If the dough is still sticking to the bowl after five minutes, add a small amount of flour, then knead until it's no longer sticky (about 30 seconds).

PACK IT UP

- Lightly flour a countertop or table and place the dough on it.
- Cut the dough into three equal pieces, then roll each one into a ball.
- Want to save the dough for later? Lightly flour each one and place it in a plastic bag in the refrigerator (for up to a day) or coat it in olive oil and freeze it (for up to three months).

READY TO MAKE PIZZA?

- Remove the dough from the fridge/freezer and let it come to room temp.
- Sprinkle flour onto a countertop or table, then use the palms of your hands to stretch the dough until it feels like it can't be stretched any further, but will still fit on your pizza stone.
- Preheat the oven to 500°F with a pizza stone on the middle rack.
- Place the dough onto a cutting board with a piece of parchment paper under the dough, then try to cut away any excess paper so it doesn't burn in the oven!
- Add sauce and toppings, then place the pizza onto the pizza stone.
- Cook until the crust is golden brown (about eight to 10 minutes), then remove from the oven using a pizza paddle or large cutting board.
- Cut, serve, and enjoy!

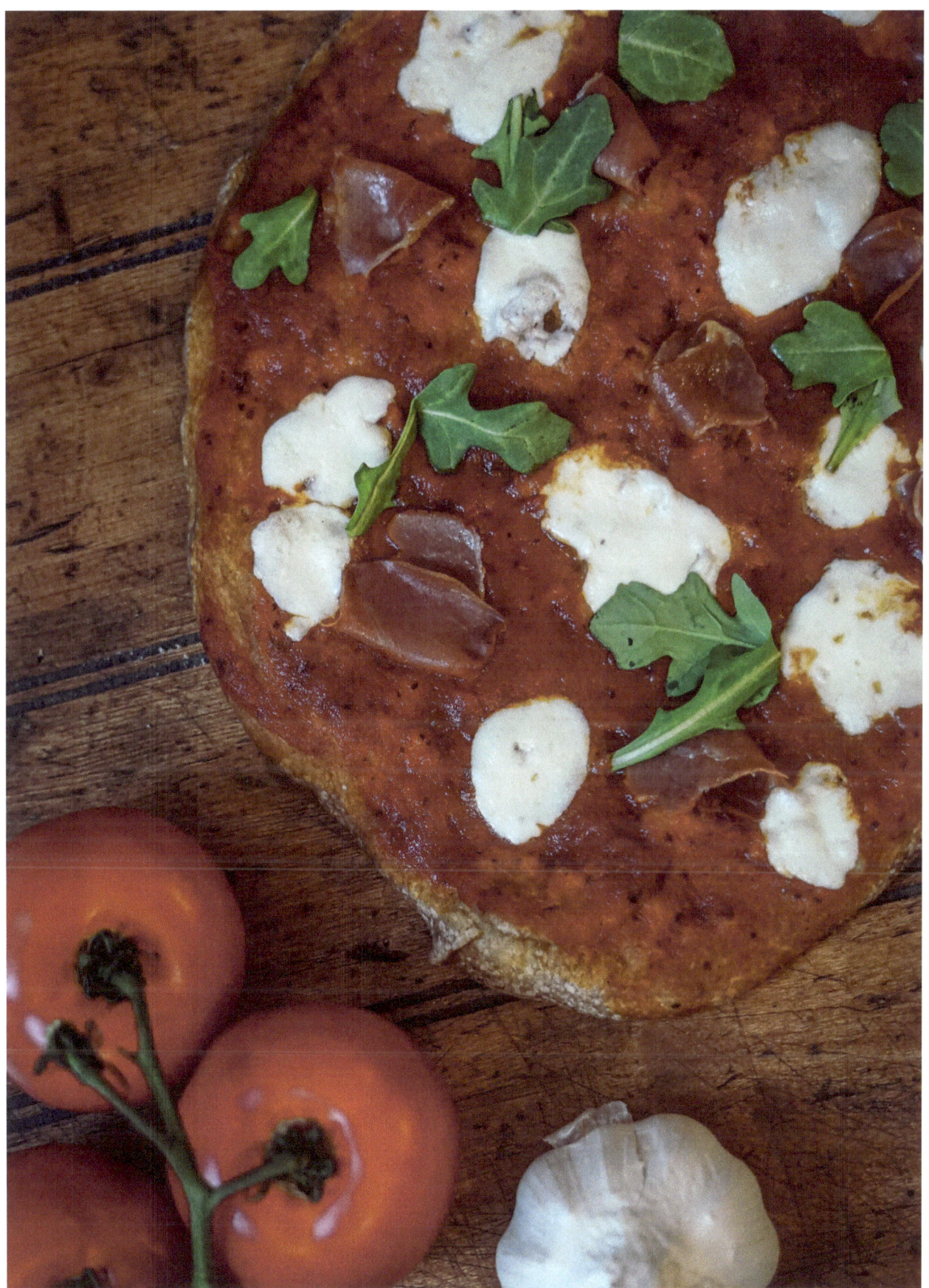

FEELING BROKE
RAMEN POPCORN $0.81

MAKES 16 CUPS
OM NOM NOM

PAIRS WELL WITH:
- FEEDING THE MASSES
- NIGHTS IN
- NIGHTS OUT

ACTIVE TIME
8 MINUTES
TOTAL TIME
10 MINUTES

SPECIAL EQUIPMENT
Large pot with lid (for stovetop)
Paper bag (for microwave)

INGREDIENTS
- 2 Tablespoons olive oil or coconut oil
- ½ cup popcorn kernels
- 2 Tablespoons melted butter, margarine, or ghee
- 1 packet ramen seasoning

SWITCH IT UP
Not feeling the ramen? Swap in another seasoning of your choice.

INSTRUCTIONS
STOVETOP
- Heat a large pot over medium heat, then add the oil.
- As the oil starts to heat up, toss a few kernels into the bottom of the pan - these are your oil temperature gauges. Once these kernels pop, the oil is hot and ready to go!
- Add the rest of your kernels, put a lid on the pot, then shift the pot around so the kernels get evenly coated in oil.
- The kernels should start popping pretty quick. Once they get going, carefully tip the lid to let steam escape from the pot, then keep shaking until there's no longer a steady pop coming from the pan.
- Remove from heat, then add the butter to the kernels.
- Shake, mix in the ramen seasoning, and enjoy!

MICROWAVE
- Put the popcorn and oil in a paper bag. Fold the top down to ensure the bag stays shut.
- Press your popcorn button, or heat on high for two minutes or so, until you don't hear steady popping any longer.
- Remove from the microwave, open the bag, add the melted butter, then fold the top of the bag back down and shake.
- Add the ramen seasoning, shake, and nom!

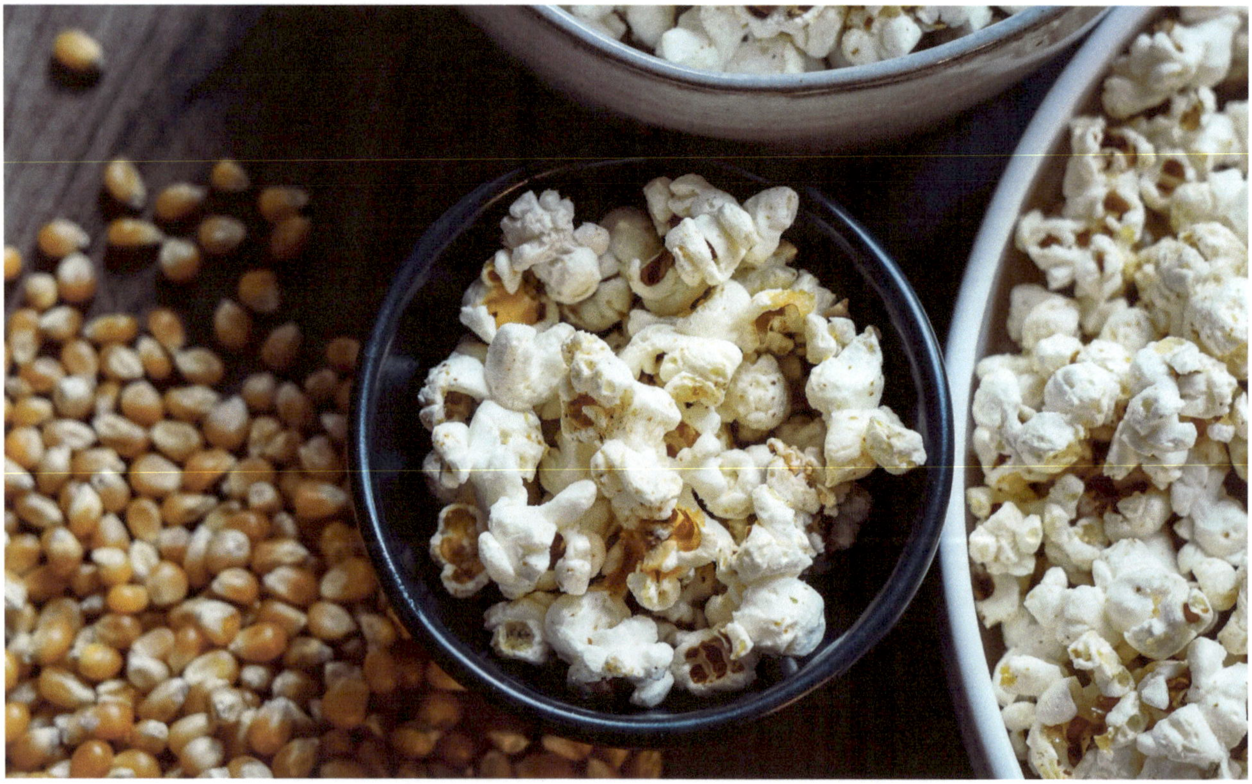

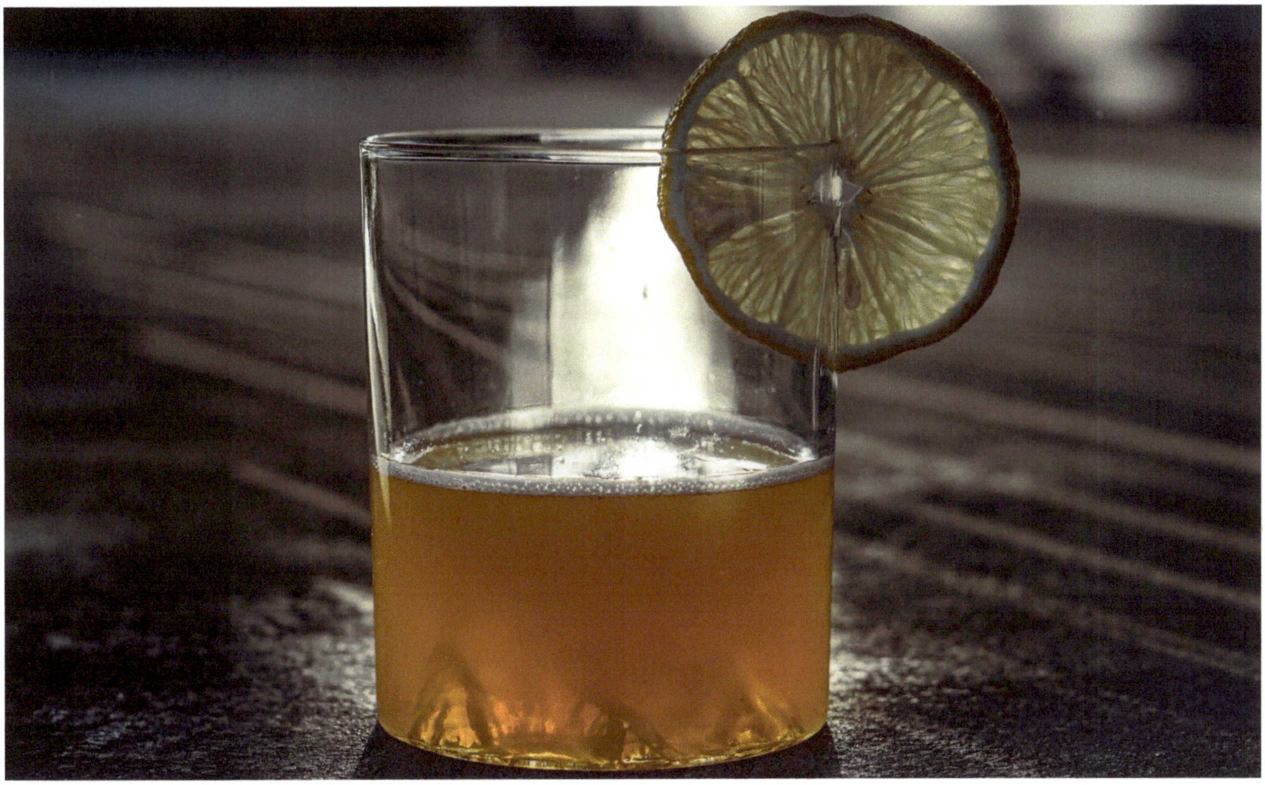

GOLD RUSH $2.50

MAKES 1 DRINK

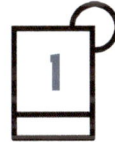

PAIRS WELL WITH:
- MIXING THINGS UP
- IMPRESSING YOUR GIRLFRIEND
- DIY GIFT GIVING

TOTAL TIME
5 MINUTES

INGREDIENTS
- ¾ ounce honey syrup (we'll teach you how to make it)
- 2 ounces bourbon
- 2 ounces lemon juice
- Lemon wedge for garnish
- Fresh ice

INSTRUCTIONS
- Start by making the honey syrup: Mix equal parts honey and water in a saucepan with the stove turned to medium.
- Stir until the honey is dissolved but not simmering (only a minute or two), then set it aside to cool.
- Put into a jar with a lid and store in the fridge.
- Pour the bourbon, lemon juice and honey syrup into a cocktail shaker. Toss in a handful of ice and shake until chilled (about 30 seconds).
- Strain the liquid into a lowball glass (or whatever you're drinking from), add a few cubes of ice, garnish with a lemon wedge, and enjoy.

FEELING

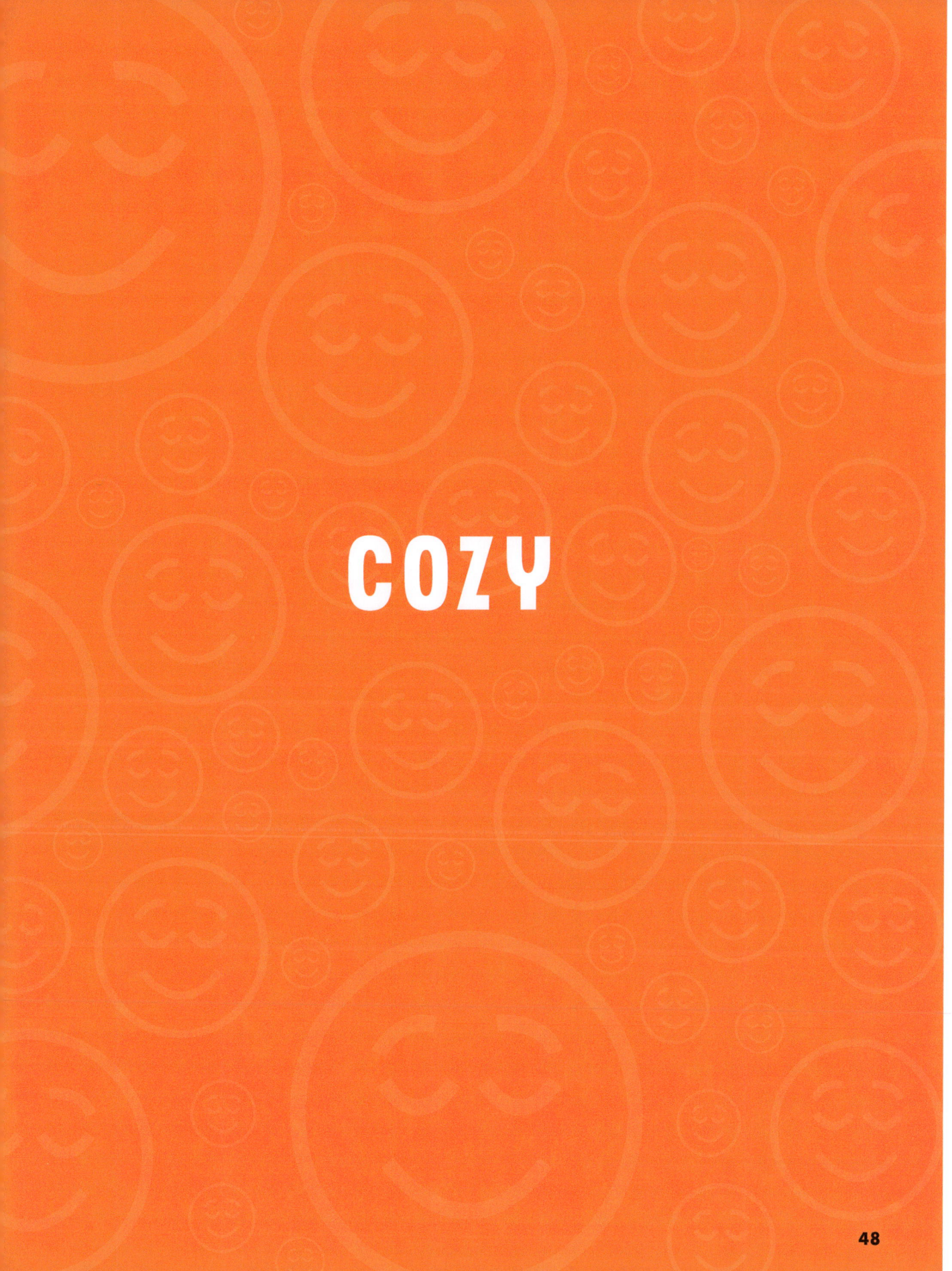

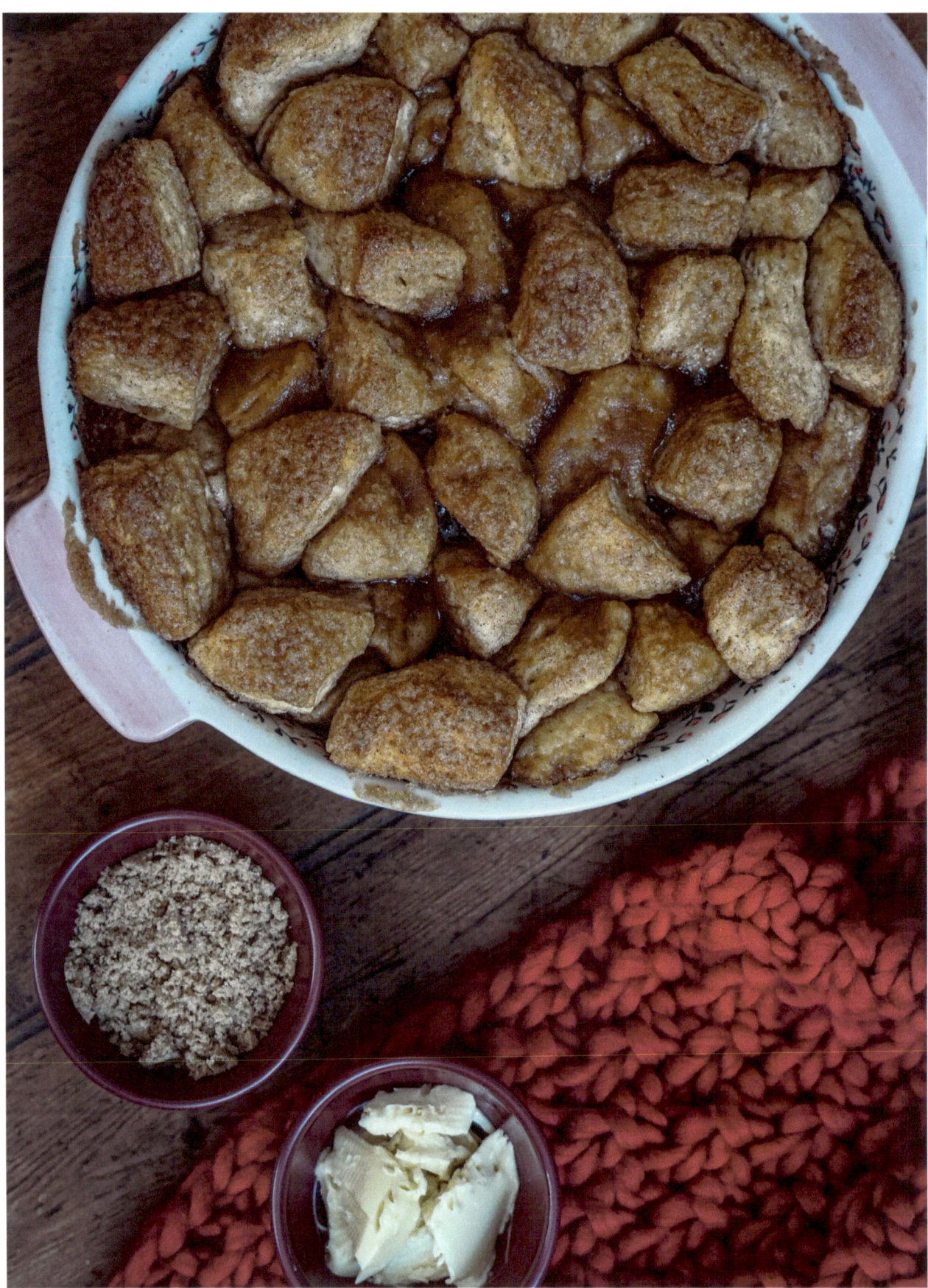

FEELING COZY

SLOW MORNING MONKEY BREAD

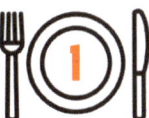

MAKES 1 PAN OF CARAMELLY BREAD CHUNKS

PAIRS WELL WITH:
- HOT COFFEE
- FUZZY CLOTHING
- BEGINNERS

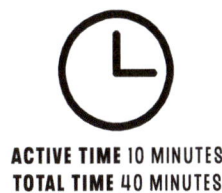

ACTIVE TIME 10 MINUTES
TOTAL TIME 40 MINUTES

INGREDIENTS

1 cup white sugar
2 teaspoons cinnamon
36 ounces refrigerated biscuit dough
¾ cup diced apple (optional)
½ cup brown sugar
1 cup butter or butter alternative
Canola oil spray

INSTRUCTIONS

Preheat the oven to 350°F and find a bundt pan, bread pan, muffin tin, or anything else that'll do the job and coat with canola oil spray.

In a large bag or bowl, mix the white sugar with the cinnamon and set it aside.

Cut all of the biscuit dough into bite-sized pieces.

Coat the biscuit chunks, a few at a time, in the cinnamon sugar and place into your pan of choice. If you're into apples, you can add them as you fill the pan. Set aside the extra cinnamon sugar, and remember: the dough will expand as it bakes, so be sure to leave a little room in the top of the pan!

In a small pot, combine the brown sugar, ⅓ cup of the remaining cinnamon sugar, and the butter. Stir the mixture as the butter melts and the sugar dissolves, then bring to a boil for one minute until it turns into a thick, caramel-y syrup.

Drizzle the syrup generously over the dough, letting it fill in the nooks and crannies in the pan.

Bake on the center rack of the oven, until the dough is light brown and crispy on the outside (about 30 minutes).

Remove the pan from the oven, let it cool, and prepare for flippage! Place a large baking sheet or plate on the top of the pan. Holding the sides of the pan tightly, flip the whole thing over to release the bread (and syrup) from the pan. If the biscuit pieces aren't cooperating, run a butter knife around the sides of the pan to release them.

Eat, then fall into a sugary nap.

FEELING COZY

PANCAKES + CINNAMON HASH

MAKES PLENTY FOR FOUR PEOPLE

PAIRS WELL WITH:
- SUNDAY MORNINGS
- AUTUMN LEAVES
- BIG FAMILIES

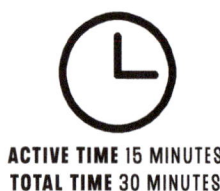

ACTIVE TIME 15 MINUTES
TOTAL TIME 30 MINUTES

SPECIAL EQUIPMENT

Griddle (optional)
Whisk

INGREDIENTS

PANCAKES

1 ½ cups flour
4 teaspoons baking powder
½ teaspoon salt
1 egg
1 ¼ cups milk
4 Tablespoons butter, melted
½ teaspoon vanilla (1 cap full)
Canola oil spray

HASH BROWNS

1 large or 2 medium sweet potatoes
½ teaspoon salt
1 teaspoon cinnamon
1 ½ Tablespoons vegetable oil

INSTRUCTIONS

THE PANCAKES

- In a large bowl, whisk together the flour, baking powder and salt.
- In another bowl, combine the egg, milk, melted butter, and vanilla.
- Create a well at the bottom of the dry mix.
- Add the wet mix into the well and fold the two mixes together until you have a generally lump-free batter. You can use a whisk if the lumps are being stubborn.
- Heat a griddle (or fry pan) over medium-low, then spray the pan with oil.
- Drop a cute little dab of batter onto the pan to make a tiny test pancake.
- Once you've confirmed the pan is hot enough with your tiny test pancake, measure out about $1/3$ cup of batter at a time into the pan. Remember to keep a bit of space between pancakes so you can flip them
- Cook each cake for two to three minutes on each side (the first side is ready to flip when you start seeing consistent bubbles forming on the top of the batter).
- Repeat until the batter is gone, then set the pancakes aside or keep them warm in the oven at a low temperature.

THE HASHBROWNS

- Peel the sweet potato, then use a large cheese grater to shred it into a bowl of ice-cold water.
- Stir the shreds gently, then drain off the cold water. This will help remove some of the potato's starch.
- Once strained, put the potato shreds onto a rimmed baking sheet and press the moisture out of them with a few paper towels or a tea towel.
- Put the potato back into the (dry) bowl and add the salt and cinnamon.
- Stir vigorously.
- Add the oil and stir to ensure all of the potato is evenly covered.
- Heat the griddle (or pan) again, spray with oil, then add your hashbrowns (in batches if needed). Cook on each side until they start to crisp up (about five minutes), then flip.
- Serve the pancakes and hashbrowns together with a heap of butter and a bathtub of syrup.

HOT TIP

Want to add chocolate chips or blueberries to your pancake batter? We like to add these right after we put the batter on the griddle. This allows you to customize each person's pancakes.

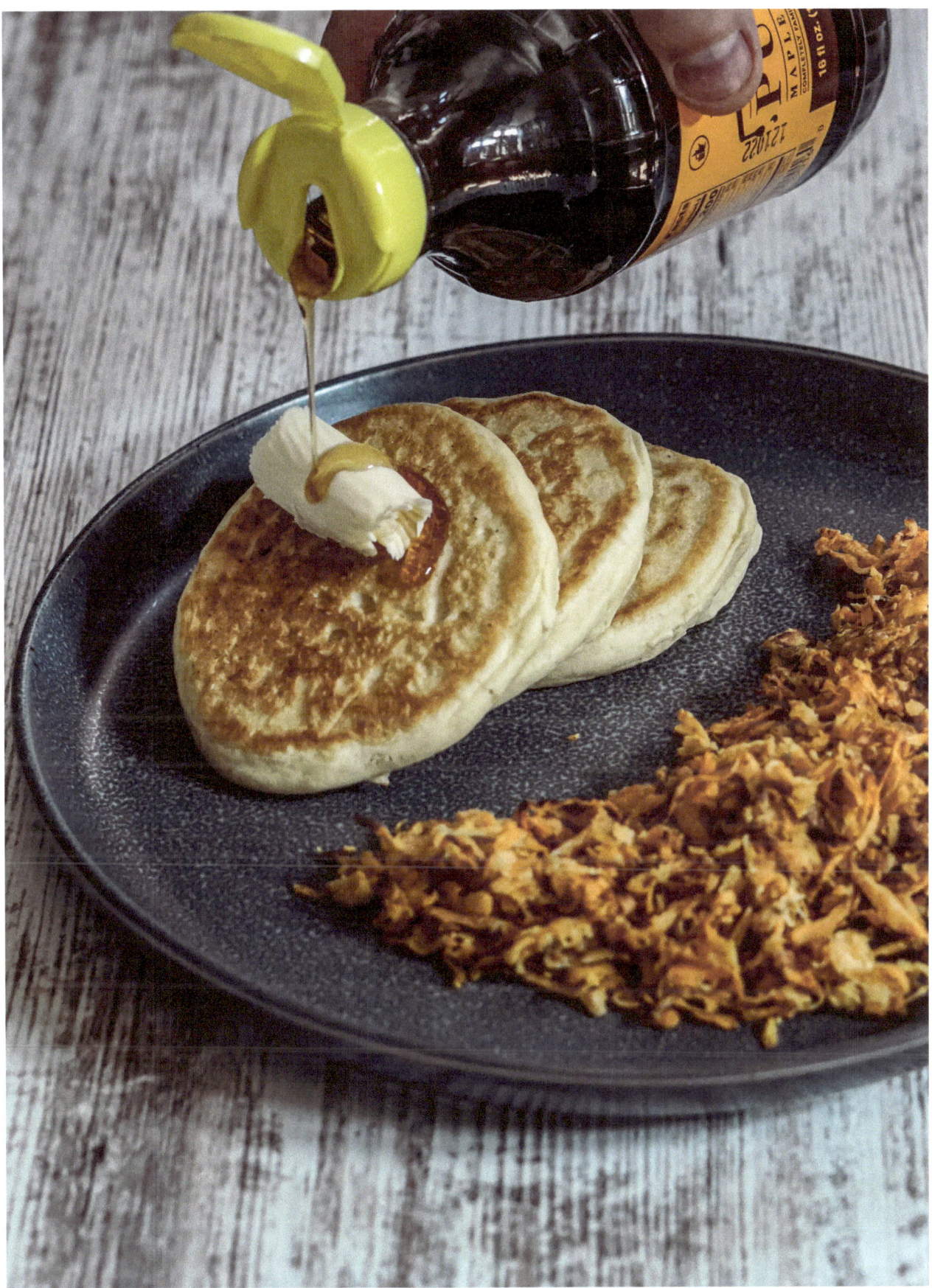

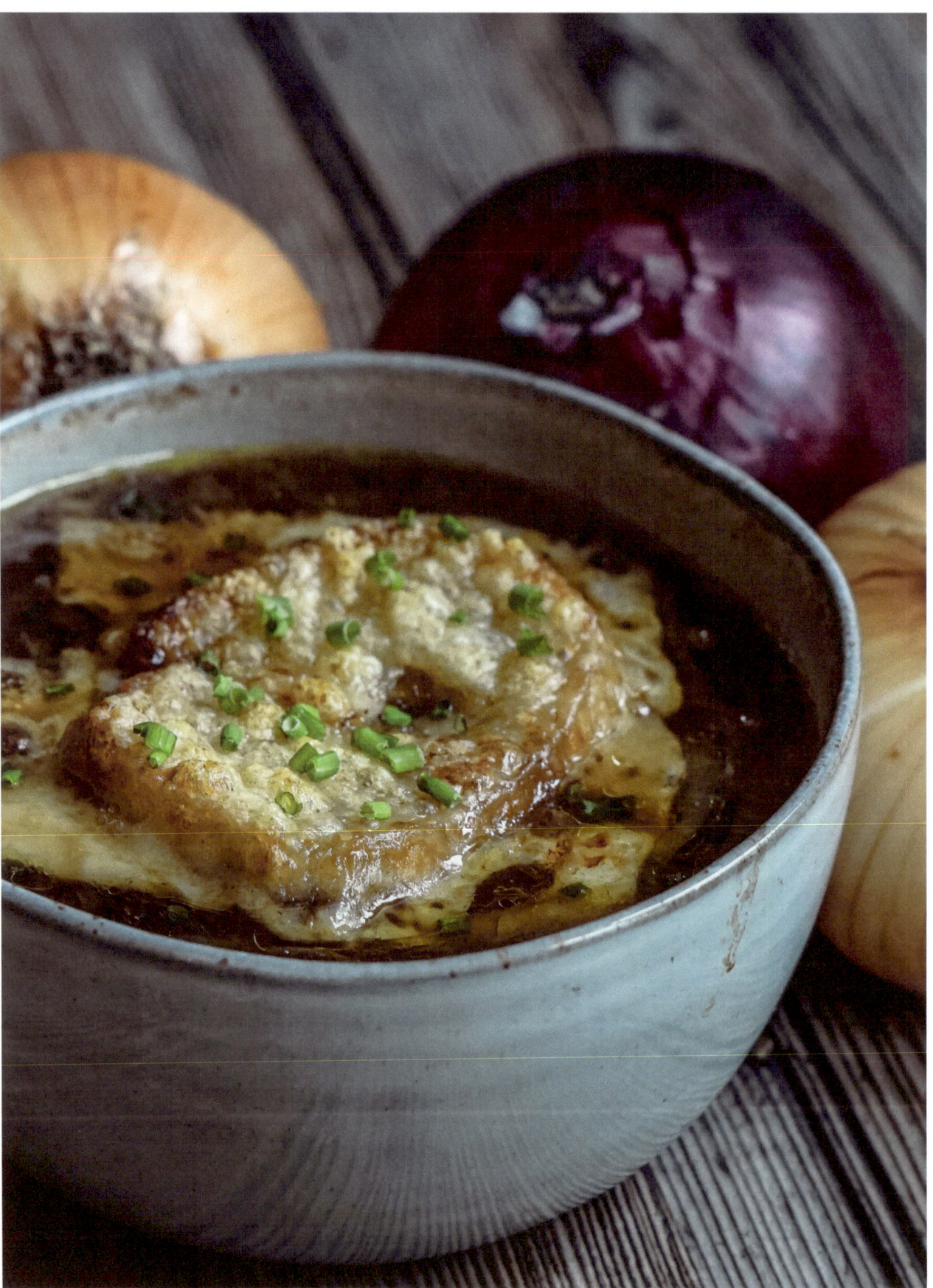

FEELING COZY

FRENCH ONION SOUP

MAKES 4 LARGE SERVINGS

PAIRS WELL WITH:
- SWEATER SEASON
- PEOPLE WHO TOLERATE SLURPING SOUNDS
- VEGETARIANS

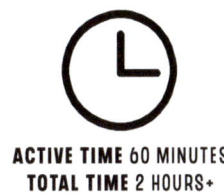

ACTIVE TIME 60 MINUTES
TOTAL TIME 2 HOURS+

SPECIAL EQUIPMENT

One large stock pot
Wooden spoon/spatula
4 oven-safe bowls or ramekins

INGREDIENTS

Patience
3-4 pounds onions (ideally 2/3 yellow, 1/3 red, and a few shallots)
1/3 cup butter or margarine
1 Tablespoon salt
1 Tablespoon pepper
1/2 cup dry sherry or vermouth
8 cups chicken stock
3 sprigs thyme
2 bay leaves
1 teaspoon fish sauce (optional but adds depth)
2 teaspoons apple cider vinegar
4+ slices french or rustic bread, toasted
3 cloves garlic, chopped
4 slices gruyere or swiss cheese
Chives, for garnish

FOR THE DETAIL ORIENTED

If you're using a plant-based butter alternative, it's possible that the onions may turn more translucent and sweet rather than a golden hue. Don't worry, they will still be delicious.

INSTRUCTIONS

Open a window. Slice all the onions and shallots into a bowl, then have yourself a good cry.

Feel better? Good. Melt the butter in a large stock pot over medium-high heat. Add the onions to the pot, splitting them into batches if they don't fit in the pot all at once.

Cook the onions, stirring occasionally, until translucent.

Turn the heat down to medium-low, and let the onions continue to cook until they turn golden (about an hour, could be longer).

Use a wooden spoon to frequently stir the onions and make sure nothing burns to the bottom of the pot. Stuff happens, so if you notice a small burnt spot, just add a touch of water, scrape it away, and keep moving.

Once the onions hit that beautiful golden state, add the salt, pepper, and sherry.
Turn the heat to medium and give the whole pot a good scrape with the wooden spoon. This will deglaze the pot and keep the cooking going nicely.

Simmer for about five minutes until the alcohol smell disappears.

Add the chicken stock, thyme, and bay leaves, and simmer for another 20 minutes. If the simmer (small bubbles) turns into a boil (big bubbles), lower the heat to keep things under control.

Pour the fish sauce and apple cider vinegar into the pot, then pull the thyme and bay leaves out.

Taste the soup and salt as needed.

Toast the bread, then spread it with garlic and keep it nearby.

Turn the broiler on and move an oven rack as needed to allow your bowls to fit in the oven. Place each bowl on a baking sheet, fill with soup, then lay the toast and cheese on top.

Broil until the cheese is melted and golden brown, then remove from the oven.

The bowls of soup will be hot at this point, so let them cool, garnish with chives, and serve!

FEELING COZY

CHICKEN POCKET PIES

MAKES ABOUT 12 POCKETS

PAIRS WELL WITH:
- BIG OL' BLANKETS
- PORTION CONTROL
- AVOIDING THE DISHES

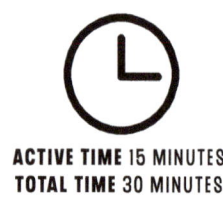

ACTIVE TIME 15 MINUTES
TOTAL TIME 30 MINUTES

SPECIAL EQUIPMENT

Parchment paper
Cooling rack (helpful but not required)

INGREDIENTS

4 sheets puff pastry, thawed
4 Tablespoons butter or butter alternative
½ of a yellow onion, diced
3 carrots, peeled and diced
3 celery stalks, diced
1 Tablespoon thyme
1 teaspoon salt
½ teaspoon pepper
3 Tablespoons flour
1 ¼ cups chicken stock
½ cup high-fat milk (we like coconut milk but cow works too)
1 ½ cups shredded chicken (of any variety)
½ cup frozen peas
1 egg
1 Tablespoon water
Nonstick cooking spray

INSTRUCTIONS

- Preheat the oven to the specified heat on the puff pastry box (usually around 400°F).
- Grab yourself a saucepan and melt the butter over medium-high heat.
- Toss in the onion, carrots and celery (mirepoix anyone?) and saute until the celery and carrots start to soften (about four or five minutes).
- Add the thyme, salt and pepper and stir to incorporate.
- Turn down the heat to medium, stir in the flour, and cook for two more minutes while you change into some sweats.
- Pour in the chicken stock and milk and stir to incorporate. The mixture should start to thicken at this point.
- Gently stir until the gravy is almost paste-like and thick enough to stick to a spoon.
- Add the chicken and peas, stir, and taste.
- Adjust the seasoning to your liking, then remove from heat and set aside while you prep the pastry.
- Sprinkle some flour onto a large cutting board or bulletproof countertop, then unroll the dough.
- Using a knife or pizza cutter, make an "X" to cut the dough into four triangle pieces.
- In a small bowl whisk together the egg and water.
- Add a spoonful of pie filling into the center of each triangle. Lightly brush the egg wash around each edge of each triangle, then fold half of the dough over the other, turning the large triangle into a smaller triangle.
- Pinch the edges together to seal, then repeat until all your pastry is used up.
- Line a baking sheet with a piece of parchment paper, then lightly cover with nonstick spray.
- Gently transfer the pastries onto the baking sheet. Be sure to leave about a finger-width of room between pieces so they have room to grow.
- Bake for about 20 minutes, until the pastry is golden brown and you can't help but smell the yummy smells.
- Remove your yummy little pockets from the oven. Unless you want to burn your face off, we recommend placing them on a cooling rack for a few minutes before serving.

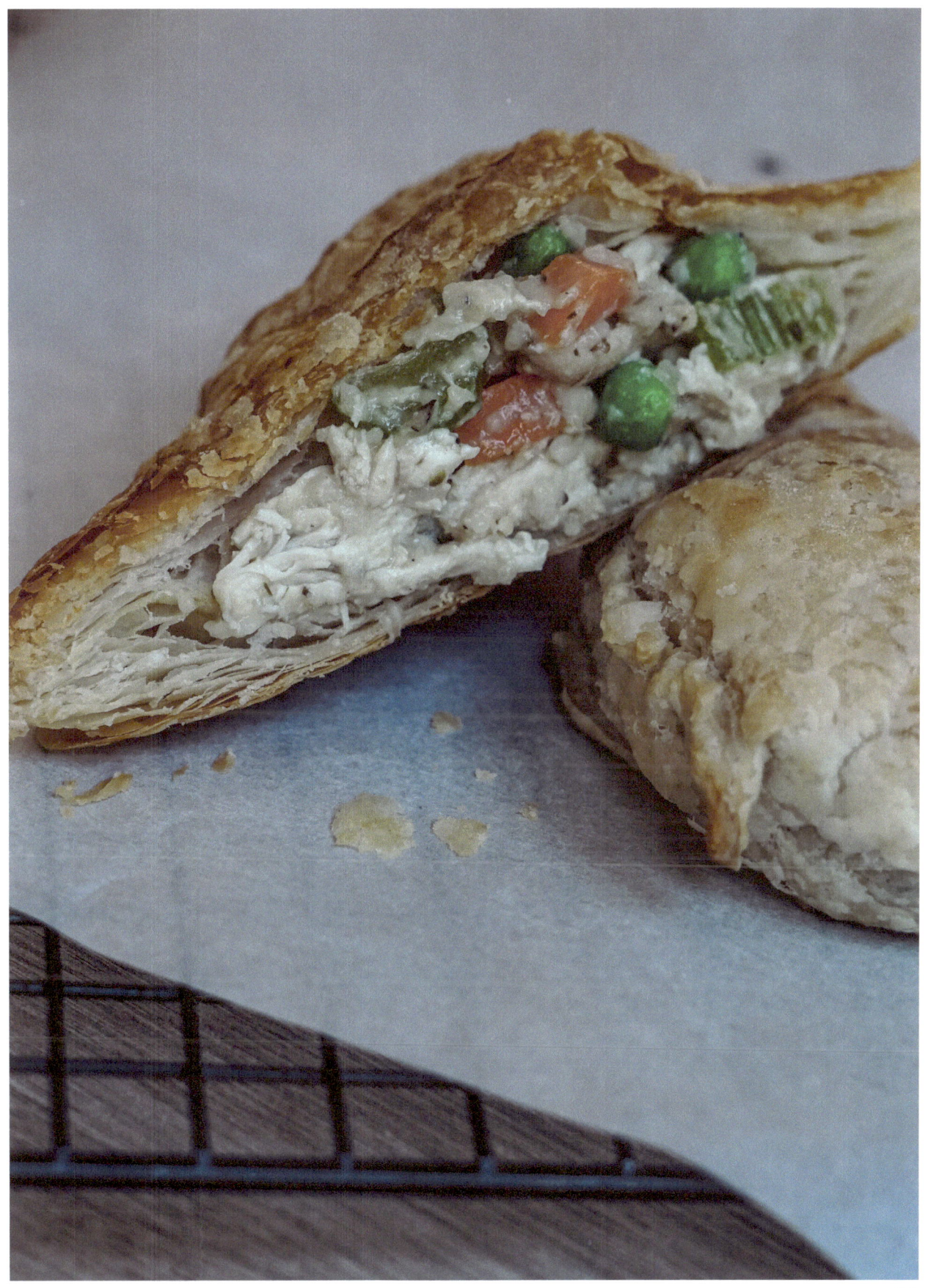

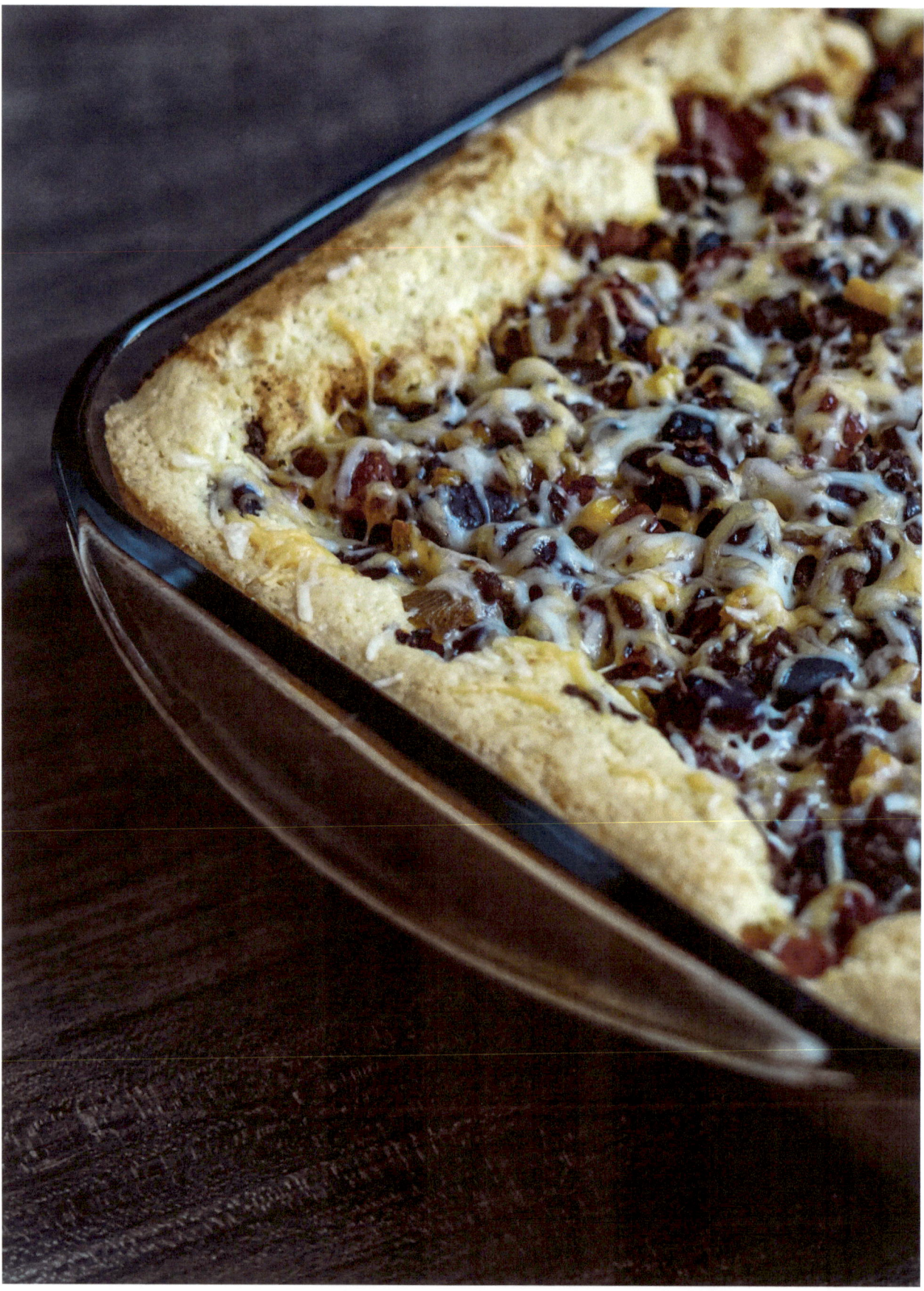

FEELING COZY

COMFY CORNBREAD CASSEROLE

MAKES 1 9X13 PAN (ABOUT 8 SERVINGSS)

PAIRS WELL WITH:
- EMPTY TUPPERWARE CONTAINERS
- SOUTHERNERS
- HONEY, HONEY

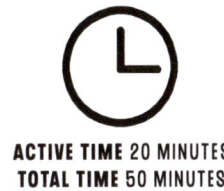

ACTIVE TIME 20 MINUTES
TOTAL TIME 50 MINUTES

SPECIAL EQUIPMENT

Stock Pot
9x13 pan
Colander or strainer

INGREDIENTS

2 boxes cornbread mix and the ingredients necessary to make them (likely milk and eggs)
1 pound ground beef (or meat substitute of choice)
1 large onion, any color
3 cloves garlic, chopped
1 can fire-roasted tomatoes
1 Tablespoon chili pepper
2 teaspoons cumin
2 teaspoons oregano
2 teaspoons salt
1 ½ teaspoons black pepper
1 can black beans, drained and rinsed
1 can kidney beans, drained and rinsed
1 can fire-roasted corn, with its juice
2 cups shredded mexican blend cheese
Green onion and cilantro for garnish, diced
Sour cream (optional)
Nonstick cooking spray

INSTRUCTIONS

Start by heating a stock pot on the stove over medium-high.

Add the ground beef. Once it starts to brown, add in the chopped onion and garlic, then use a spatula to stir the pot until the beef is fully cooked and the onions are translucent.

Strain the fat off into a small dish, set aside to cool, then transfer the beefy mixture back into the stock pot.

Turn the heat down to medium and add the tomatoes to the pot.

Give the mixture a quick stir, then add the chili powder, cumin, oregano, salt, and pepper. Let this cook for about five minutes, stirring occasionally, until it's giving off a nice aroma.

Add the black beans, kidney beans and corn. Stir again (we really like stirring), then turn to low and simmer while you work on the cornbread.

Preheat the oven to 375°F.

Spray a 9"x13" with cooking spray. Follow the box directions on the cornbread to make the mix, then pour the batter into the pan, using a spatula to push it into an even layer.

Gently pour the stock pot of deliciousness onto the layer of cornbread, being intentional to leave a little bit of cornbread "crust" around the entire dish.

Get that thing in the oven before you overthink it, and bake for about 20 minutes. Pull the pan out of the oven, cover the chili in cheese, and return to the oven until the cornbread is cooked (golden-brown) and the cheese is nice and melty.

Remove it from the oven, garnish with green onion, cilantro, and a dollop of sour cream.

Claim the best spot on the couch and enjoy!

FEELING COZY

GRANDMA MURRAY'S BEEF STEW

MAKES 12 BOWLS

PAIRS WELL WITH:
- MINNESOTA WINTERS
- CRUSTY BREAD
- AN EMPTY FREEZER

ACTIVE TIME
15 MINUTES
TOTAL TIME
4.5 HOURS

SPECIAL EQUIPMENT
Large, oven-safe stock pot and lid
Meat thermometer

INGREDIENTS
- 2 pounds beef stew meat
- 3 celery stalks, chopped
- 3 carrots, peeled and chopped
- 5 medium potatoes, peeled and cubed
- 2 medium onions, chopped
- 2 slices bread, broken
- 1 Tablespoon sugar
- 4 cloves garlic, diced
- 2 - 14 ounce cans of crushed tomatoes
- ½ can water

INSTRUCTIONS
- Preheat the oven to 250°F.
- Mix all ingredients together in a large stock pot and salt generously.
- Cook until the internal temp of the meat is between 160°F and 180°F and the potatoes are tender (about 4.5 hours).
- Add salt and pepper to taste and enjoy.

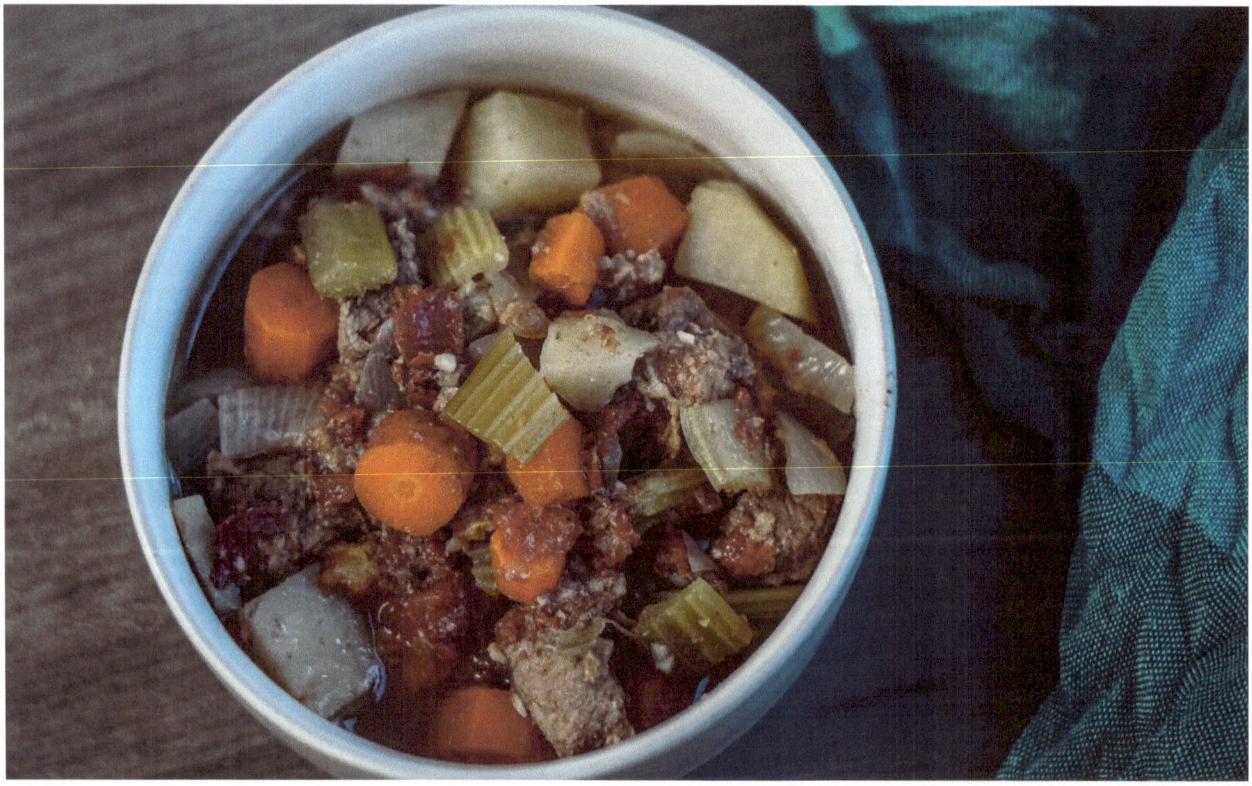

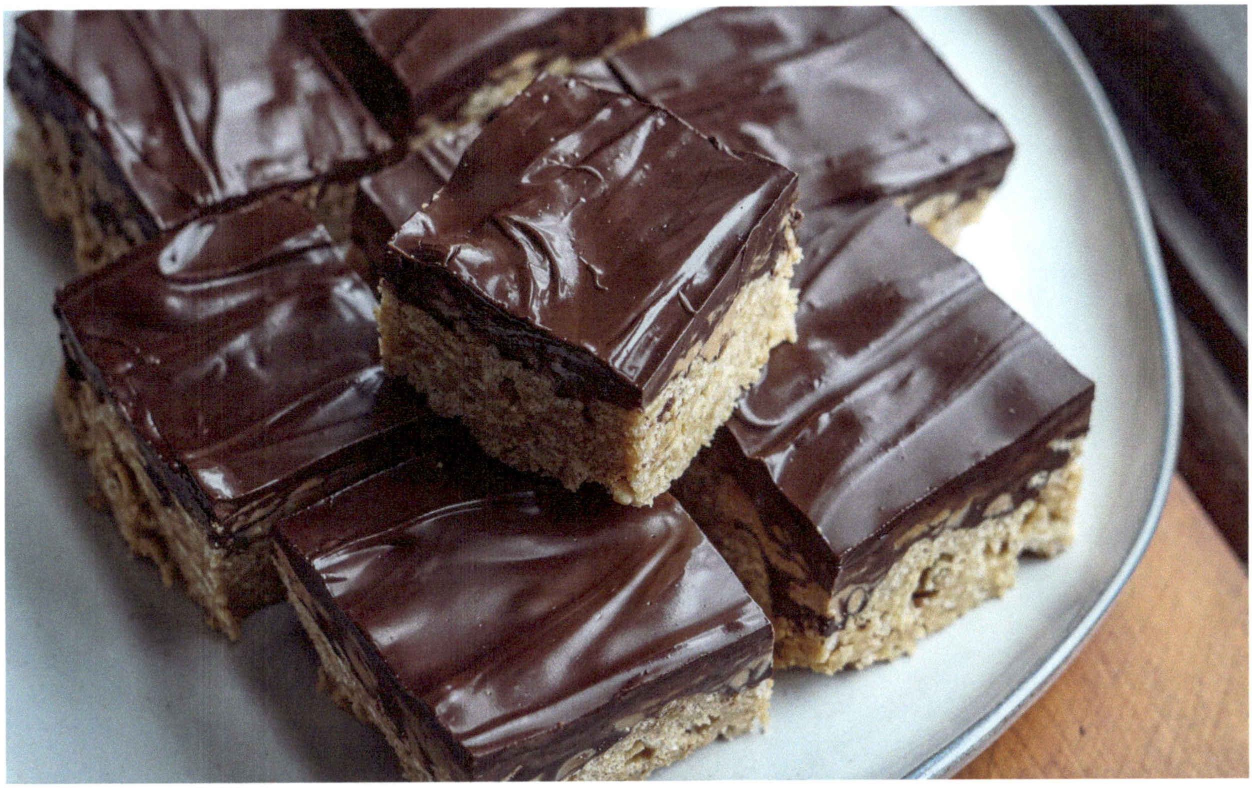

SPECIAL K BARS

MAKES 1 PAN (ABOUT 12 SERVINGS)

PAIRS WELL WITH:
- SHOWING AUNT KAREN WHO'S BOSS
- SUGAR CRAVINGS
- GATHERINGS

ACTIVE TIME
10 MINUTES
TOTAL TIME
20 MINUTES

SPECIAL EQUIPMENT
9x13 glass baking dish

INGREDIENTS
- 6 cups Special K cereal
- 1 cup sugar
- 1 cup corn syrup
- 1 teaspoon vanilla
- 1 cup creamy peanut butter
- 1 bag chocolate chips
- 1 bag butterscotch or peanut butter chips

INSTRUCTIONS
- Preheat the oven to 350°F, then grease a 9x13 dish.
- Measure the cereal into a large bowl and set aside.
- In a medium saucepan, combine the sugar and corn syrup and bring to a rolling boil.
- Remove from heat, add the vanilla and peanut butter, and stir until creamy.
- Pour the mixture over the cereal and fold until evenly distributed.
- Transfer the contents of the bowl into the greased 9x13 pan, then use a spatula to level out the mixture.
- Sprinkle the chocolate and butterscotch chips across the surface of the gooey goodness.
- Bake until the chips are soft and shiny (about three to five minutes).
- Remove from the oven and use a spatula to spread the chips into a smooth, even layer over the top of the mixture, combining as you go to make one solid color on top. If you happen to misplace your spatula at this step in the process, a tongue works surprisingly well.

FEELING COZY

UPGRADED TOMATO SOUP + GRILLED CHEESE

MAKES 2 SOUP + SANDWICH SETS

PAIRS WELL WITH:
- A GOOD CRY
- AN EMPTY PANTRY
- JAMMIES

TOTAL TIME 20 MINUTES

SPECIAL EQUIPMENT

Griddle (or substitute a fry pan on the stove)

INGREDIENTS

GRILLED CHEESE
4 Tablespoons mayo
4 slices brioche bread
2 slices sharp cheddar cheese
4 slices brie cheese

SOUP
1 can tomato soup
1 can full of water
2 Tablespoons fresh rosemary
¼ cup sour cream
6 leaves fresh basil

INSTRUCTIONS

GRILLED CHEESE

Set the griddle to a medium heat setting.

Spread one tablespoon of mayo onto both sides of each slice of bread, being sure to keep the bread slices separated so they don't stick together.

Place all of the freshly mayo-d bread onto the griddle.

Once they reach a golden-brown color, use a spatula to flip them over.

Layer the cheddar and brie onto half the slices, then top with a second slice from the griddle.

Once the bottom is golden-brown, flip each sandwich over and cook until the bread is golden and the cheese is melted (about two minutes).

SOUP

Pour the can of soup and a can-full of water into a pot over medium heat.

Chop the rosemary and add it to the pot.

Once the soup is nice and hot, turn the heat off, then slowly whisk in the sour cream.

Ladle into bowls, garnish with fresh basil, and serve alongside your freshly grilled cheese sandwiches.

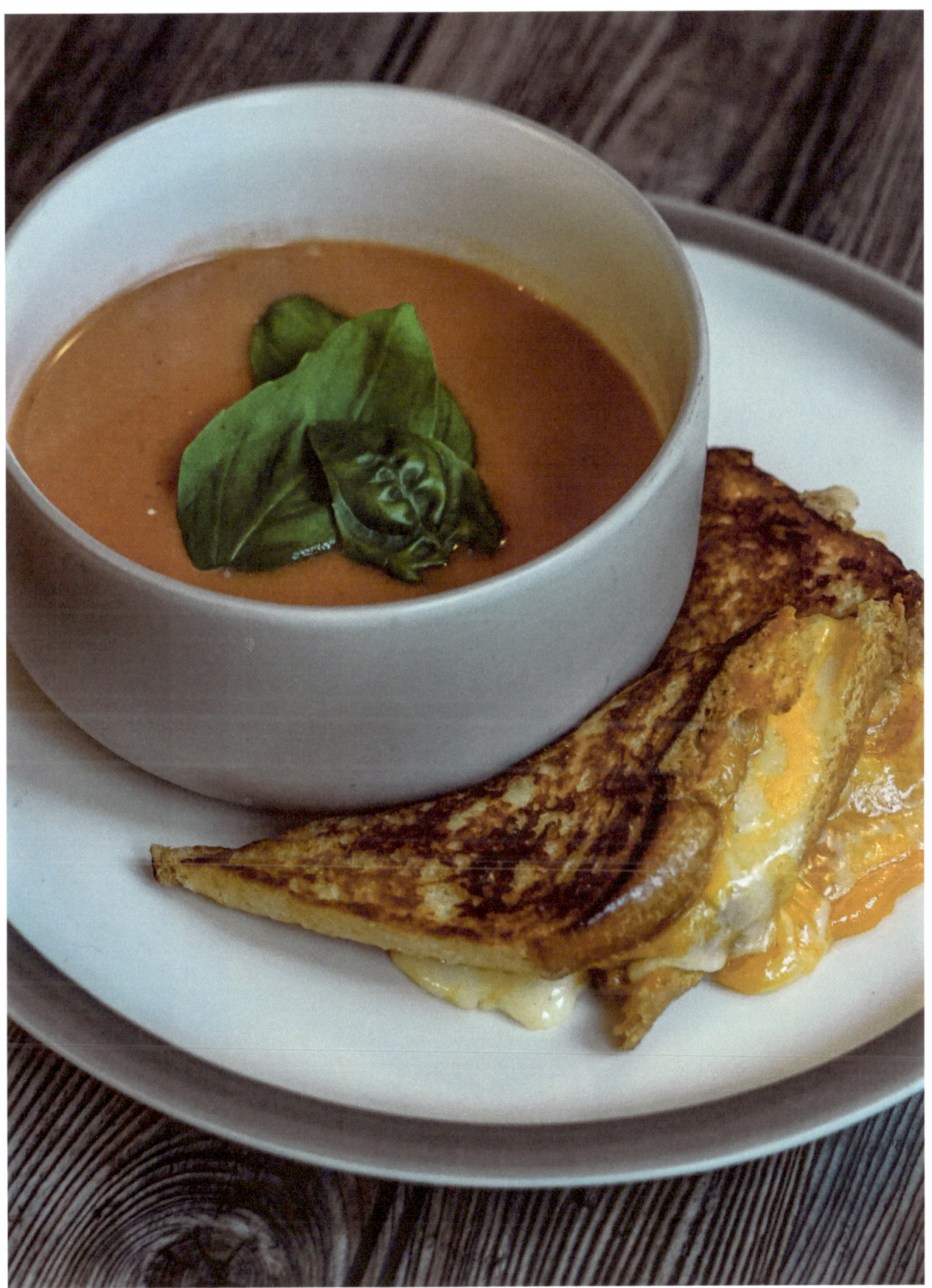

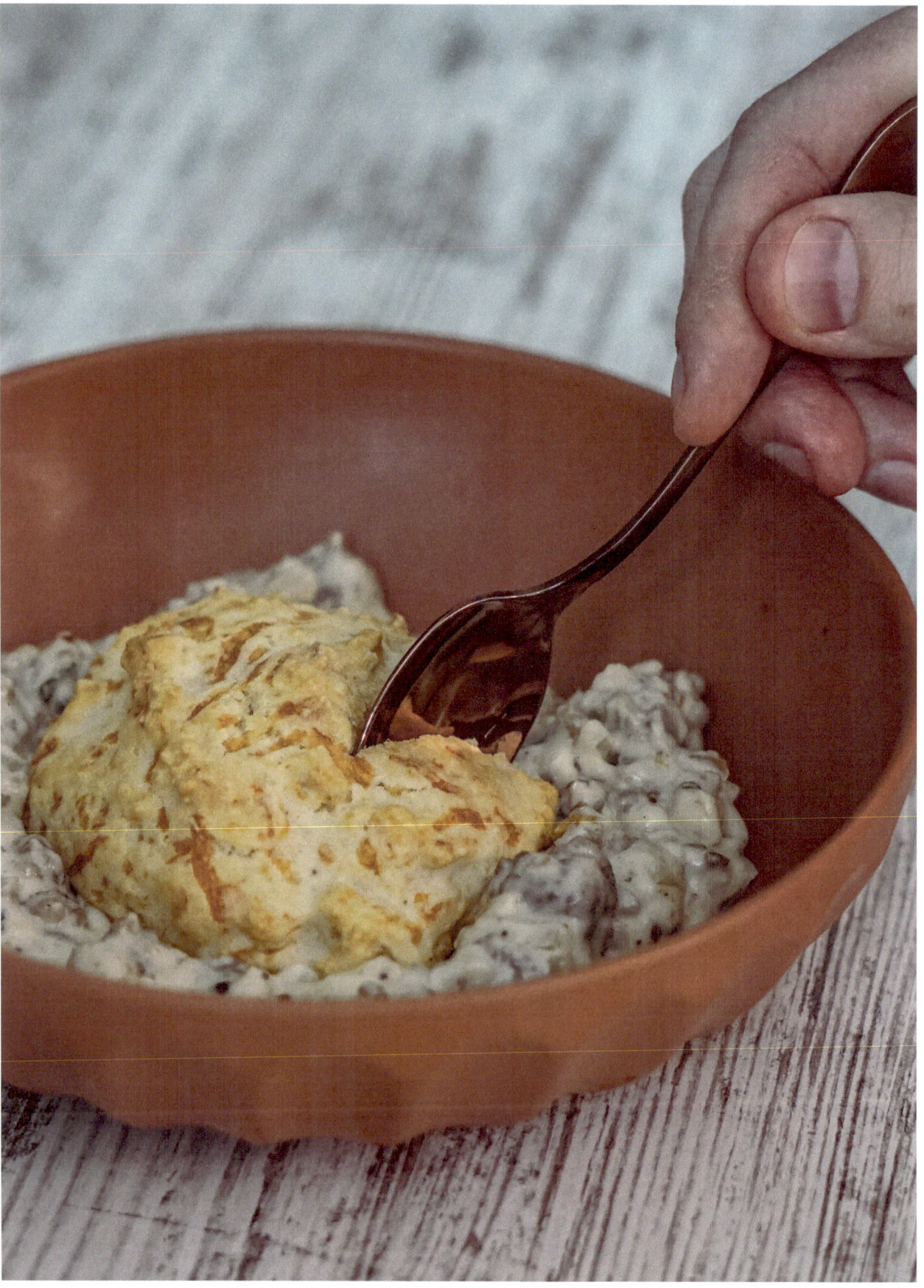

FEELING COZY

CHEDDAR BISCUITS & GRAVY

MAKES 10 BISCUITS + 5 BOWLS

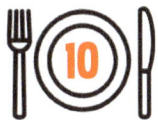

PAIRS WELL WITH:
- LONG NAPS
- COLD DAYS
- FIREPLACES

TOTAL TIME 30 MINUTES

INGREDIENTS

1 box cheddar bay biscuits (available at most grocery stores)
1 pound pork sausage
4 Tablespoon butter or butter alternative
1 medium sweet onion, diced
3 cloves garlic, minced
¼ cup flour
2 cups half-and-half or coconut milk
2 chicken bouillon cubes, crushed
1 teaspoon dried oregano
1 teaspoon dried thyme
½ teaspoon cayenne pepper
1 Tablespoon worcestershire sauce
Salt and pepper to taste

HERE'S THE DEAL

This recipe is super indulgent and so satisfying. Make it for a hungover brunch, a cozy night in, or whenever you're craving a savory hug of a meal.

INSTRUCTIONS

Start by making the biscuits. Follow the box directions but don't worry about the garlic butter.

When the biscuits are in the oven, brown the pork sausage in a deep-sided pan over medium heat, using a firm spatula to break it into crumbles. Once browned, pull the sausage out of the pan, drain off any fat, and set aside.

Return the empty pan to the burner. Add the butter and the onions, cooking until the onions are soft and translucent. Add the garlic and cook until the room fills with yummy smells (about one minute).

Now for the hard part! SLOWLY add the flour to the pan while stirring constantly. Once the flour is fully incorporated into the onions, cook for another minute, until the flour has slightly browned.

Stir in the half-and-half about a half-cup at a time.

Once the half-and-half is fully incorporated, toss in the boullion, oregano, thyme, and cayenne. Does it look like a sauce now? Great! Add the worcestershire sauce, salt and pepper to taste, then fold in the sausage.

Ding! The biscuits are done, and now, so is the gravy. Put one on top of the other (your call) and serve.

FEELING COZY
MELLOW MASH

MAKES 1 HECK OF A BOWL

PAIRS WELL WITH:
- WEIGHTED BLANKETS
- ROMANTIC COMEDIES
- LONG WEEKS

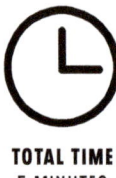

TOTAL TIME
5 MINUTES

INGREDIENTS
- 1 box instant mashed potatoes
- 2 Tablespoons butter
- 1 spoonful sour cream
- 1 sprig chopped green onions
- Bacon bits
- Salt and pepper, to taste

HERE'S THE DEAL
My wife/co-author loves me most, but mashed potatoes are a close second. During cold or rainy days, she'll pull out the instant potatoes, turn on the kettle, and nestle up on the couch.

-Rob

We've added a few touches to the recipe to maximize yumminess, however, a little butter and salt go a long way.

INSTRUCTIONS
- Boil water. Measure out the amount recommended by the directions on the box and pour into the bowl of the pre-measured potatoes.
- Stir in the butter and sour cream.
- Add the green onions, bacon bits, salt, and pepper to taste.
- Hand to your loved one who's too cozy to get up.

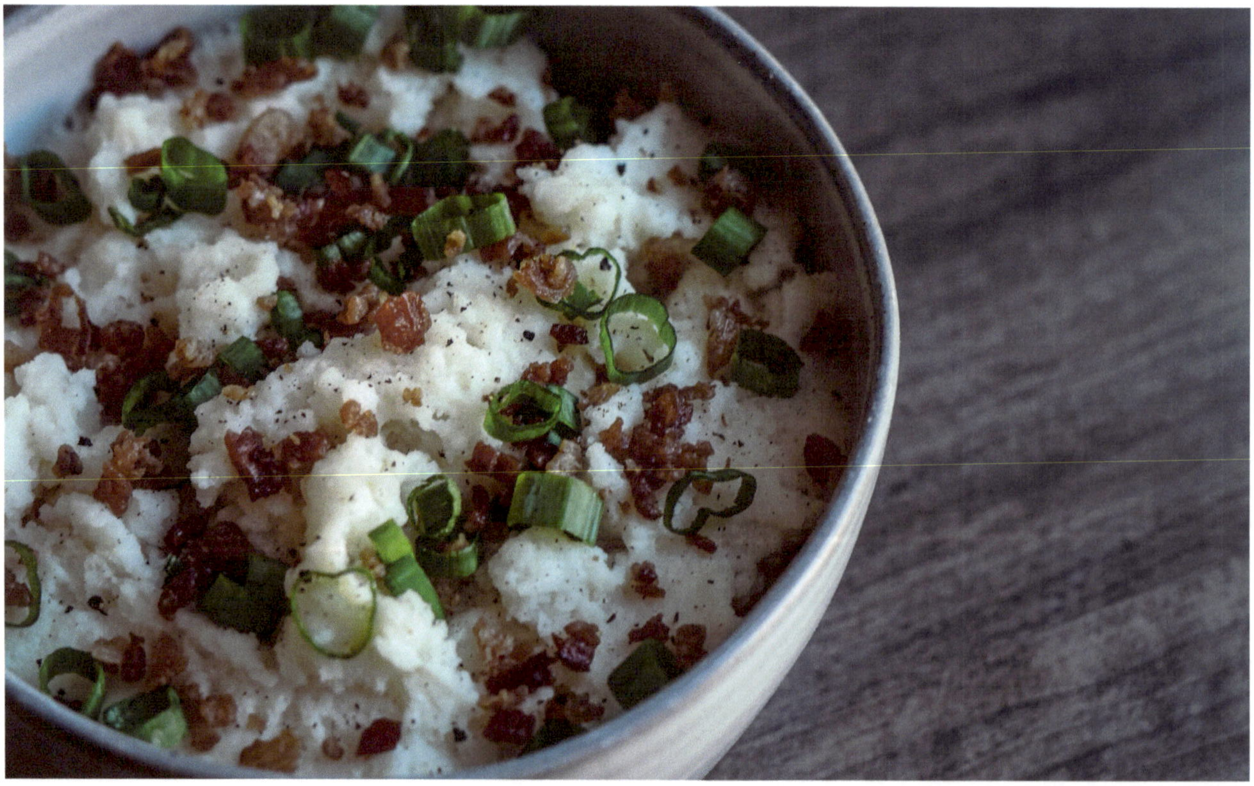

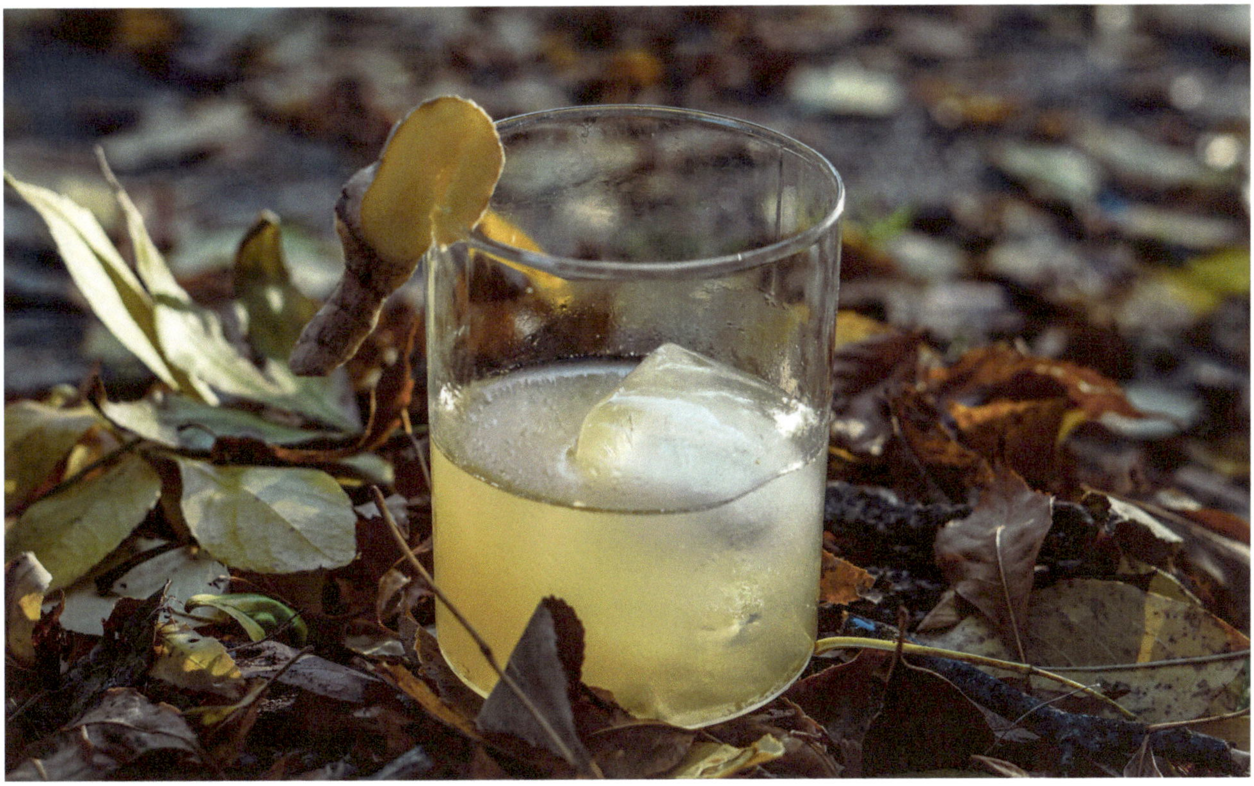

PENICILLIN

MAKES 1 DRINK

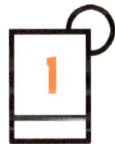

PAIRS WELL WITH:
- PAINFUL CONVERSATIONS
- PEOPLE WHO THINK THEY DON'T LIKE SCOTCH
- GINGER BEER GEEKS

TOTAL TIME
3 MINUTES

INGREDIENTS
- ¾ ounce honey syrup
- 4 thin slices of ginger
- 2 ounces blended scotch
- 1 ounce freshly squeezed lemon juice
- Fresh ice
- ½ ounce single malt scotch
- Lemon peel or ginger for garnish

A LITTLE EXTRA WARMTH
Pour the half-ounce of single malt scotch into the glass, using the back of a spoon to "diffuse" it into a thin layer on the top of each cocktail.

INSTRUCTIONS

THE HONEY SYRUP
- Mix equal parts honey and water in a small saucepan over medium heat. You want the mixture to get warm, but don't let it boil!
- Stir until the honey dissolves, then set aside to cool.

THE BODY
- Place the ginger slices into a cocktail shaker.
- Using a muddler (or something dull that can reach the bottom of the shaker), mash the ginger until the juice and oils are released (about 15-30 seconds), but stop before things get too pulpy.
- Add the blended scotch, lemon juice and honey syrup into the shaker, top with a handful of ice, and shake until everything is cold and well-mixed (about 30 seconds).
- Strain into a glass over a few cubes of ice.
- Garnish with lemon peel or ginger slice and serve!

FEELING COZY
CLASSIC OLD FASHIONED

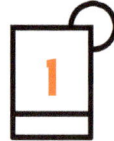

MAKES 1 DRINK

INGREDIENTS
- ½ ounce simple syrup
- 2 dashes Angostura bitters
- 2 ounces rye or bourbon
- 1 fresh orange peel (organic is best)
- 1 Maraschino cherry
- Ice

PAIRS WELL WITH:
- NIGHTCAPS
- CONFIDENCE
- BOUGIE FRIENDS

INSTRUCTIONS
- Combine the simple syrup and bitters in a short glass.
- Pour the bourbon into the glass and stir vigorously.
- Add a few cubes of ice to the glass and stir.
- Run the orange peel around the rim of the glass, then slide it down the side of the glass.
- Toss in a cherry and enjoy!

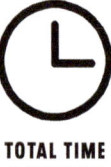

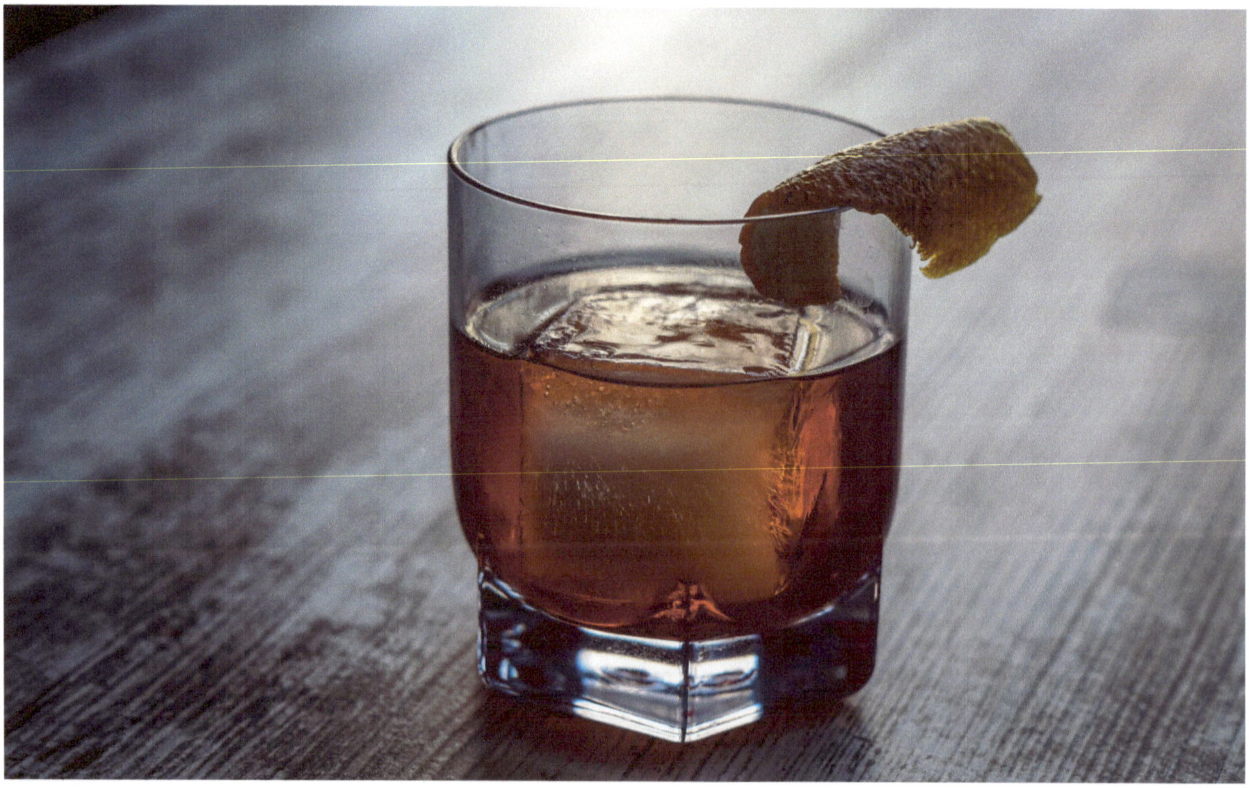

TOTAL TIME
2 MINUTES

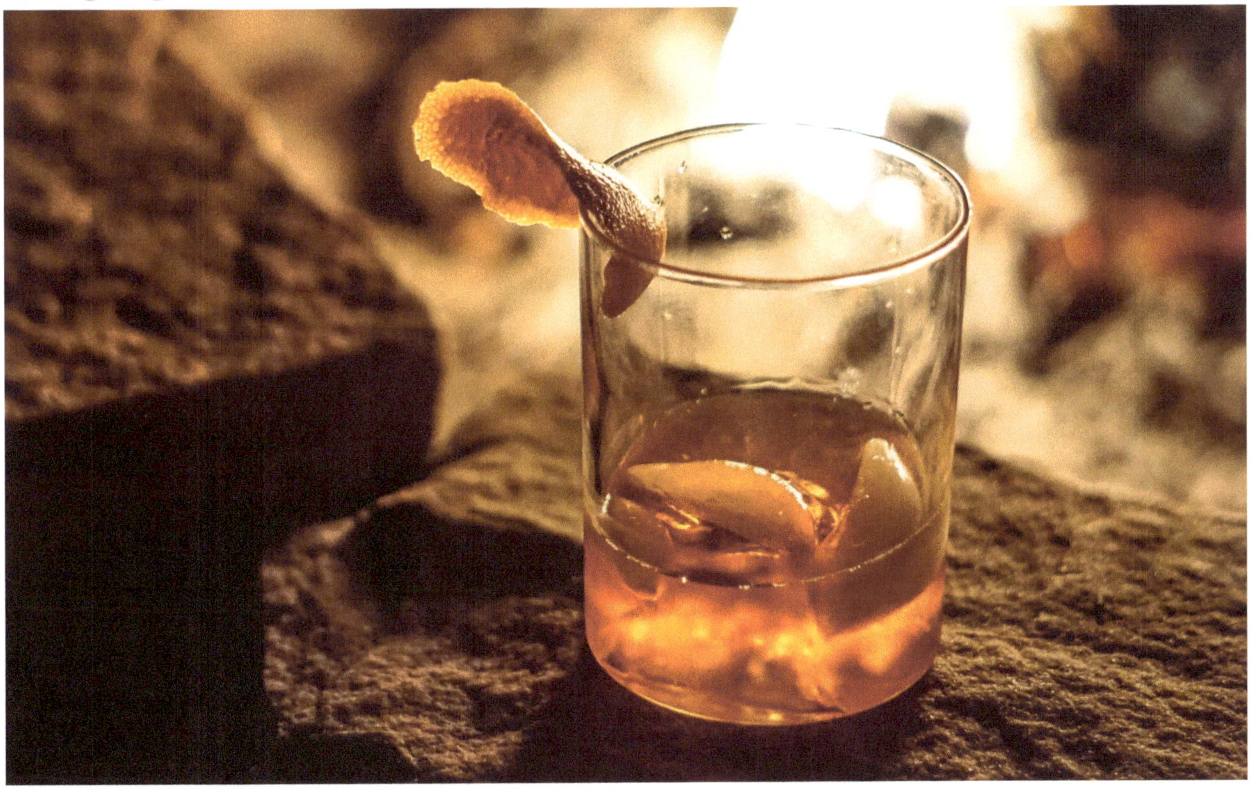

CAMPFIRE OLD-FASHIONED

MAKES 1 DRINK

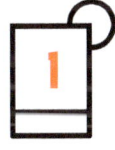

PAIRS WELL WITH:
- AFTER PARTIES
- LATE NIGHTS
- SECRETS

TOTAL TIME
2 MINUTES

INGREDIENTS
- Lemon peel (organic is best)
- 3 dashes Angostura bitters
- 3 dashes black walnut bitters
- ½ ounce simple syrup
- 2 ounces rye
- Fresh ice
- 1 Maraschino cherry

INSTRUCTIONS
- Grab the lemon peel and twist it to spray a little lemon juice into a cocktail glass of choice, then run it around the rim.
- Toss the peel into the glass, then add the bitters, simple syrup, rye and ice.
- Stir well (20 times, according to a friendly bartender in D.C.), add a cherry, and enjoy.

FEELING

FLIRTY

FEELING FLIRTY

TANTALIZING TIRAMISU

MAKES 16 SERVINGS

PAIRS WELL WITH:
- SHARING A SPOON
- YESTERDAY'S COFFEE
- WINE AND CHEESE

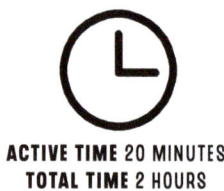

ACTIVE TIME 20 MINUTES
TOTAL TIME 2 HOURS

SPECIAL EQUIPMENT

Stand or hand mixer

INGREDIENTS

5 eggs, separated
1 cup sugar
16 ounces mascarpone cheese
2 packages lady fingers (usually in the cookie aisle)
12 ounces espresso or day-old coffee, cold
3 Tablespoons Frangelico or Kahlua liquor (optional)
Unsweetened cocoa powder
Dark or milk chocolate, for garnish

INSTRUCTIONS

MAKE THE BASE

Divide the egg whites from the yolks into two bowls.

Add the sugar to the egg-yolk bowl and whisk until creamy.

Add the mascarpone cheese and mix until smooth.

Using a stand mixer, whisk the egg whites until fluffy. We recommend gradually increasing the speed of the mixer as more air gets incorporated - if you go too fast too soon, you may end up with egg all over your kitchen. And your face.

Once the egg whites thicken and start to form stiff peaks, gently fold them into the mascarpone/egg yolk mix.

ASSEMBLY

Take an 8x8 pan, bowls, coffee mugs, or whatever you want to put this fancy dessert into, and pour a thin layer of mascarpone cream into the bottom.

Dip the lady fingers into the coffee (or coffee/liquor mixture), place across the top of the mascarpone mixture, and dust with cocoa powder.

That's one layer. Repeat a second time, then finish with any remaining mascarpone.

Chill the tiramisu in the fridge for a couple hours, then dust with cocoa and grated chocolate prior to serving.

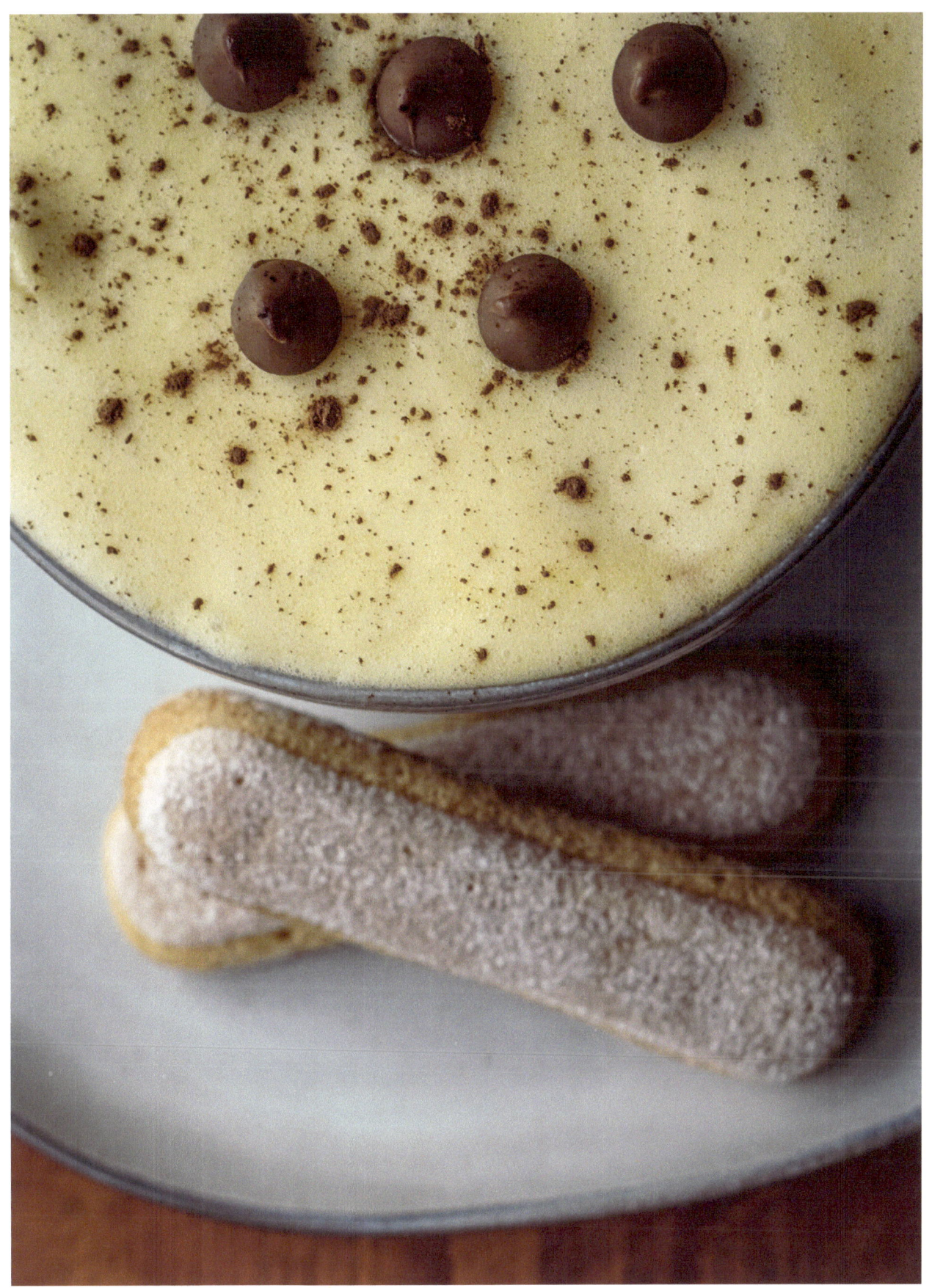

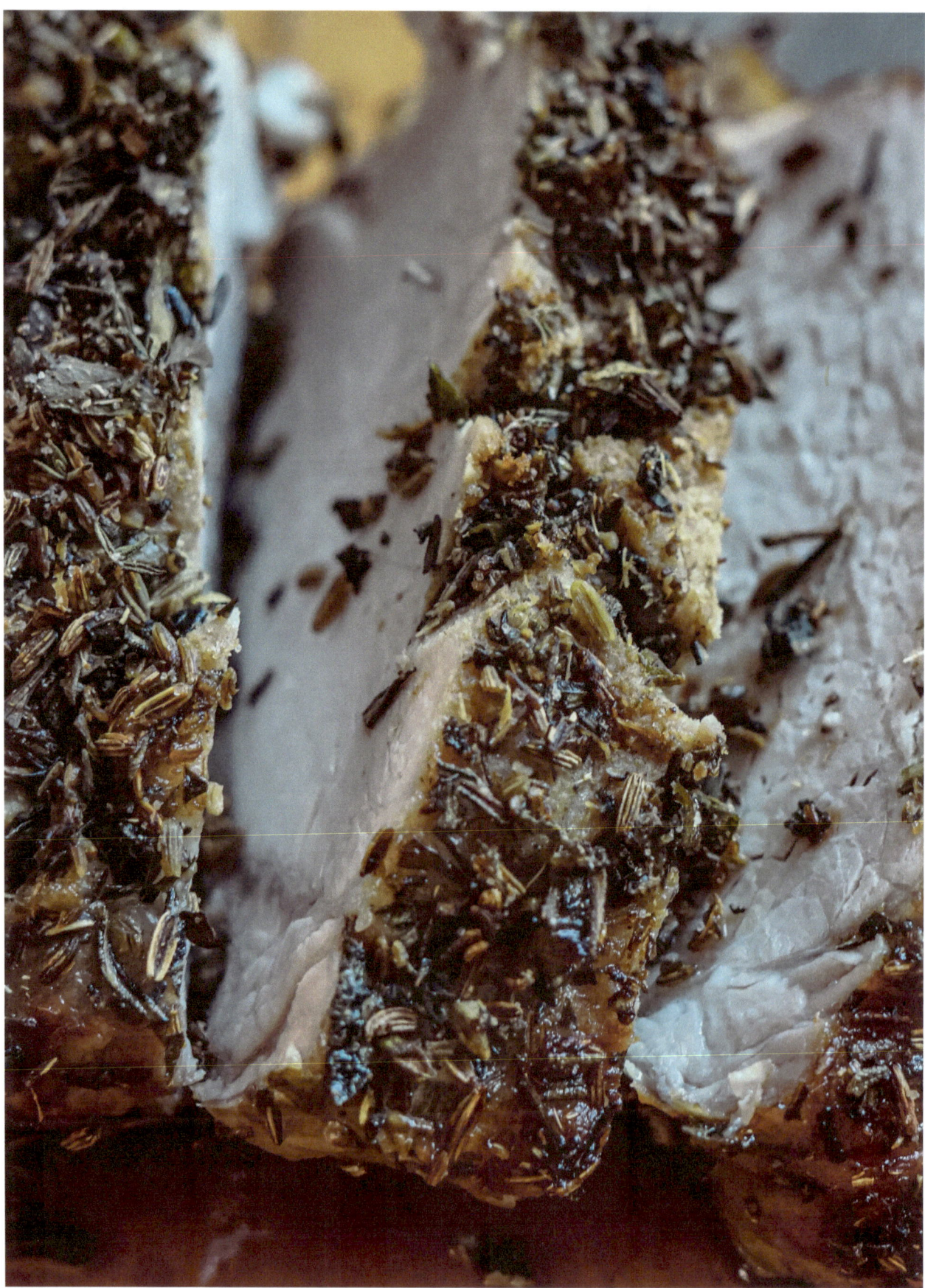

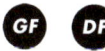

FEELING FLIRTY

MY PLACE PORKETTA

MAKES ABOUT 10 SERVINGS

PAIRS WELL WITH:
- HOT DATES
- POTATOES IN ANY FORM
- A FRESHLY STOCKED SPICE CABINET

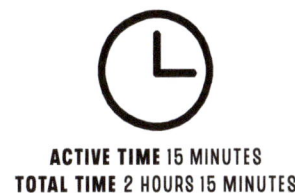

ACTIVE TIME 15 MINUTES
TOTAL TIME 2 HOURS 15 MINUTES

SPECIAL EQUIPMENT

Roasting pan
Meat thermometer
Mortar and pestle (optional)

INGREDIENTS

2-3 pounds pork loin
3 Tablespoons fennel seeds
2 Tablespoons fresh sage
2 Tablespoons fresh rosemary, minced
2 Tablespoons fresh thyme, minced
2 Tablespoons fresh parsley, minced
½ teaspoon lemon zest (this is the hardest part of this recipe)
6 cloves garlic, chopped
2 Tablespoons salt

INSTRUCTIONS

Preheat your oven to 375°F.

Start by scoring the pork loin in a diagonal pattern, making 1 inch squares across its surface.

Next, toss the fennel seeds in a small pan over medium heat and toast until fragrant (about two minutes).

Take the seeds out of the pan and grind finely in a mortar and pestle. If you don't have a mortar and pestle, chop the seeds finely.

Mix the fennel with the sage, rosemary, thyme, parsley, lemon zest, garlic, and salt.

Rub this seasoning generously all over the pork loin, place into a roasting pan, and put it in the oven until the internal temperature is 145°F (usually about two hours).
If the pork hasn't reached temp after two hours, continue cooking, checking every 10 minutes or more frequently as it gets close. Once the internal temperature reaches 145°F, turn the oven up to 450°F and cook for an additional 15 minutes until the skin is crispy (this step amps up the "yum" but is completely optional).

Remove the pork from the oven, let it rest for 15-30 minutes, then cut into ½ inch slices and serve!

Feeling Flirty

SWEETHEART-WORTHY STUFFED SHELLS

MAKES ABOUT 4 SERVINGS

PAIRS WELL WITH:
- PRETTY DISHES
- OLD SCHOOL ROMANCE
- PLANT-BASED DATES

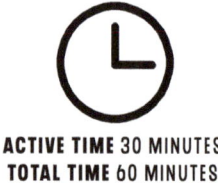

ACTIVE TIME 30 MINUTES
TOTAL TIME 60 MINUTES

SPECIAL EQUIPMENT

Blender
Heavy objects (for pressing the tofu to remove moisture)
Strainer/colander

INGREDIENTS

SQUASH SAUCE

1 large butternut squash
8 ounces jumbo pasta shells
⅓ cup cream or coconut cream
½ teaspoon oregano
½ teaspoon thyme
1 teaspoon salt
1 cup chicken or veggie broth

FILLING

1 Tablespoon olive oil
½ red or sweet onion, diced
2 cloves garlic, minced
1 pound Italian sausage (animal or plant-based)
3 cups spinach, chopped
1 cup extra firm tofu, pressed
½ teaspoon lemon zest
½ teaspoon red pepper flakes
½ teaspoon thyme
½ teaspoon oregano
½ cup cream or coconut cream
1 teaspoon salt
½ teaspoon pepper
⅓ cup parmesan, grated (optional)

INSTRUCTIONS

PREP THE SQUASH AND PASTA

Preheat the oven to 350°F. Cut the squash in half and scoop out the seeds and guts.

Line a baking sheet with parchment paper, then put the cut squash face-down on the sheet and bake in the middle rack until you can easily puncture the skin with a fork (about 30-40 minutes).
As the squash cooks, bring a large pot of water to a boil and add a tablespoon of salt.

Gently put the shells into the boiling water, then turn down the heat to medium and cook until the shells are cooked but firm. Strain and run the shells under cool water to prevent any further cooking, then set aside.

Remove the squash from the oven, let it cool until you can handle it without playing "hot potato," then scoop the squash out of its shell, into the blender.

Add the cream, oregano, thyme, salt, and broth. Blend until smooth and well combined.

MAKE THE FILLING

In a large pan, warm the olive oil over medium heat. Add the diced onion and cook until translucent (a few minutes), then add the garlic.

As the kitchen starts to smell nice and garlicky, crumble the sausage into the pan. Once the sausage is fully cooked, strain the mixture to remove any excess grease, then return it to the pan.

Gradually add the spinach. As the spinach wilts, it will shrink in size and be easier to stir into the sausage mixture. Transfer the mixture into a large bowl and set aside.

In a smaller bowl, use your (clean) hands to crumble the tofu. Add the lemon zest, red pepper, thyme, oregano and cream, then mix well.

Combine the sausage and the tofu mixtures into one bowl. Season with salt and pepper.

With the oven preheated to 350°F, pour the squash sauce into the bottom of an oven safe dish. Using a spoon (or your hands for more fun), fill the shells with the sausage mixture and place into the freshly sauced pan. Sprinkle it with parmesan if you wish, then into the oven it goes.

Bake for 15-20 minutes, serve, and enjoy.

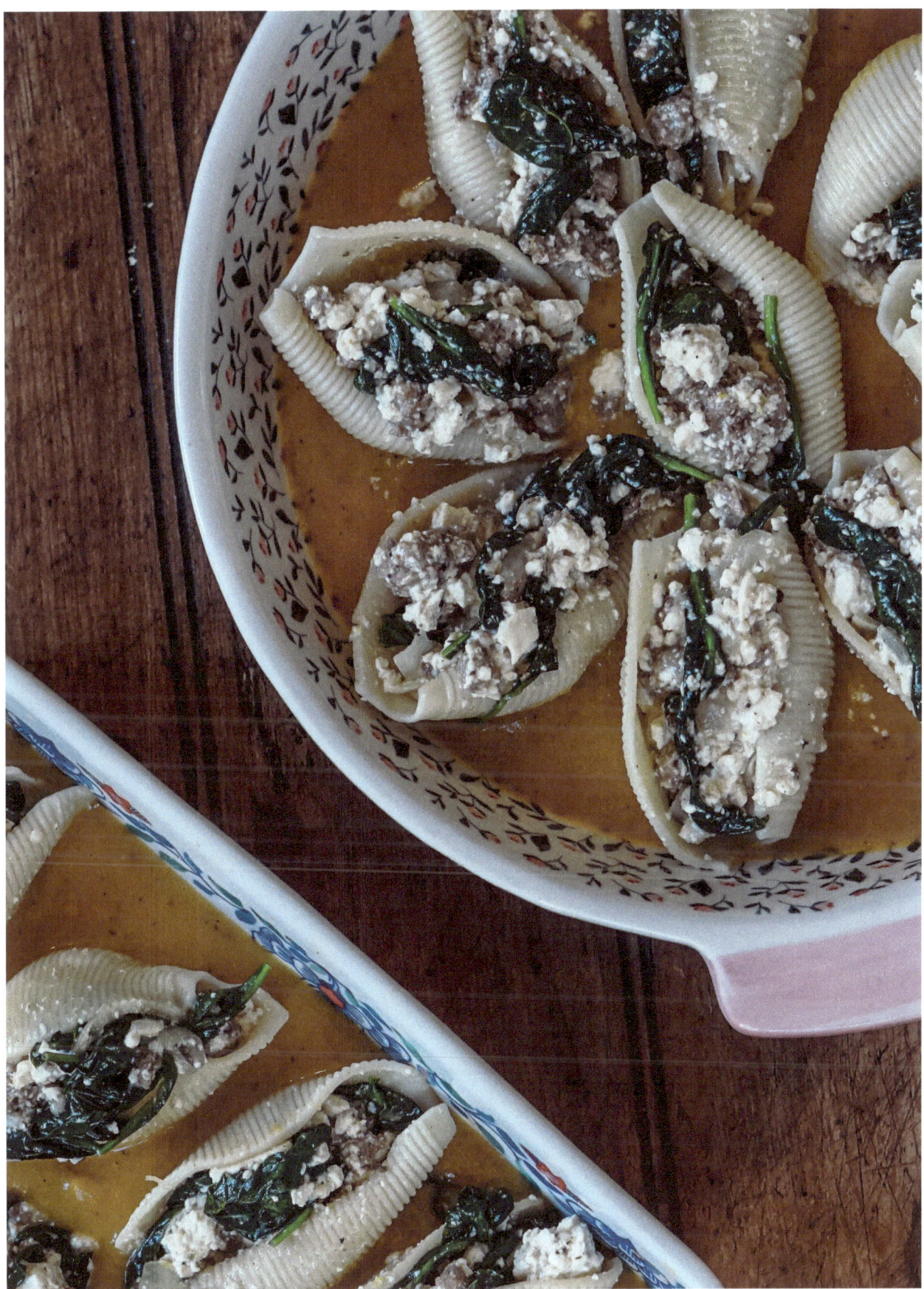

76

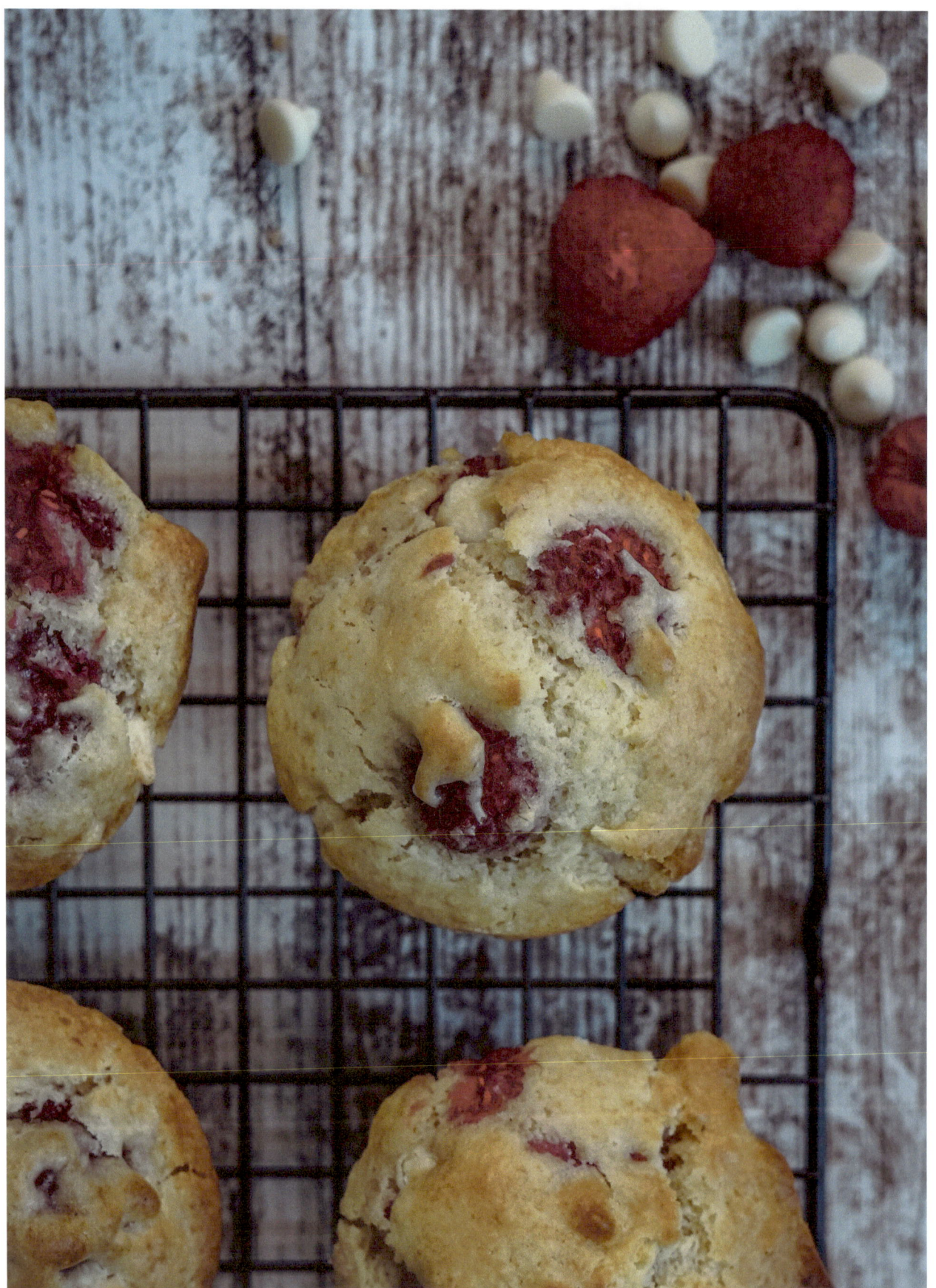

RASPBERRY WHITE CHOCOLATE MUFFINS

FEELING FLIRTY

MAKES 12 MUFFINS

PAIRS WELL WITH:
- BLACK COFFEE
- OVERNIGHT GUESTS
- LATE STARTS

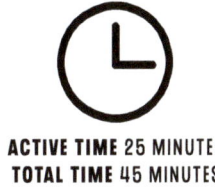

ACTIVE TIME 25 MINUTES
TOTAL TIME 45 MINUTES

SPECIAL EQUIPMENT

Cheese grater
Muffin tin liners (optional)
Pastry cutter (optional)

INGREDIENTS

MUFFINS
¾ cup milk (of any variety)
¼ cup melted butter or margarine
1 egg
½ cup white sugar
1 teaspoon vanilla
2 cups flour
2 teaspoon baking powder
½ teaspoon salt
1 cup fresh raspberries
½ cup white chocolate chips

CRUMB TOPPING (OPTIONAL)
3 Tablespoons butter or margarine
2 Tablespoons white sugar
2 Tablespoons brown sugar
⅓ cup flour

INSTRUCTIONS

PREP
Preheat your hot box (also known as an oven) to 375°F.

Grease your muffin tin or put in some fancy little muffin papers.

Whisk together the milk, butter, egg, sugar and vanilla.

In a separate bowl combine the flour, baking powder and salt.

Gently fold the dry mix into the wet using a spatula. Be careful not to overwork the mixture, as this will result in dense muffins.

Put the raspberries into a dry bowl. Sprinkle about two tablespoons of flour over the berries and shake until they look freshly sunscreeened. This flour coating will help keep them suspended in the dough while they bake instead of falling to the bottom.

Gently fold the berries and white chocolate chips into the dough, then fill your muffin tins about ¾ full with batter.

FEELING CRUMBY?
I's time to make the crumb topping! Not feeling it? Skip to the last step and bake.

Use a cheese grater to grate the butter into a bowl, then add the white sugar, brown sugar, and flour. Use the pastry cutter to combine the ingredients until they create nice little crumblies.

Add the crumblies to the top of each muffin before baking, or eat with a spoon while you watch the muffins bake. It's your kitchen.

BAKE 'EM
Bake the muffins until a toothpick inserted into the center of a muffin comes out clean (about 12-15 minutes).

Enjoy with butter, coffee, or a full brunchy spread.

FEELING FLIRTY

BOTH WAYS DEVILED EGGS

MAKES 12 EGGS
(24 BITES)

PAIRS WELL WITH:
- HOLDING HANDS
- FINGER FOOD FANATICS
- DELICATE DELIGHTS

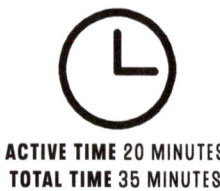

ACTIVE TIME 20 MINUTES
TOTAL TIME 35 MINUTES

SPECIAL EQUIPMENT

Blender (optional)

INGREDIENTS

TRADITIONAL DEVILED EGGS

12 eggs
½ cup mayo
2 Tablespoons dijon mustard
2 Tablespoons dill pickle relish
2 Tablespoons chives, chopped
Salt and pepper to taste

AVOCADO DEVILED EGGS

12 eggs
2 ripe avocados, pits removed
2 Tablespoons lemon juice
Zest from 2 lemons
¼ cup cilantro, chopped
Salt and pepper to taste
¼ cup chives, chopped
½ teaspoon cayenne
1 Tablespoon bacon bits

INSTRUCTIONS

Kick things off by adding the eggs to a large pot of water. Bring to a boil, then let the eggs simmer for 10-12 minutes.

At the 8 minute mark, fill a large bowl with ice water.

Remove the eggs from the pot using tongs or a slotted spoon and place them in the ice bath for an additional 10 minutes.

Once chilled, roll each egg on the counter (for the optimal humpty dumpty situation). Once the egg shell has been thoroughly cracked, peel it away and rinse the egg off to remove any lingering shell fragments.

Cut each egg in half.
Use a spoon to gently scoop the yolk out and place it in a medium-sized bowl, then set the egg white halves aside (you can immediately place them on a large plate or serving tray to save some time).

Choose your own egg adventure: Traditional or Avocado. Feel free to add either mixture to a blender for a smoother consistency.

TRADITIONAL:
Mash all the egg yolks together until smooth.
Add the mayo, dijon mustard, and relish, then mix until well incorporated.
Taste and add salt or pepper as needed.

AVOCADO:
Mash all the egg yolks together until smooth.
Add the avocado, lemon juice, lemon zest, and cilantro.
Taste and add salt or pepper as needed.

Once you are happy with the consistency, scoop the mix into a ziplock bag using a spatula. Push the mix into one of the corners of the bag, press the air out, and seal it shut. Clip a small piece of the corner off and squeeze the filling into the bowl of each egg white.

Once each egg white is filled, sprinkle with chopped chives, cayenne, bacon bits and serve.

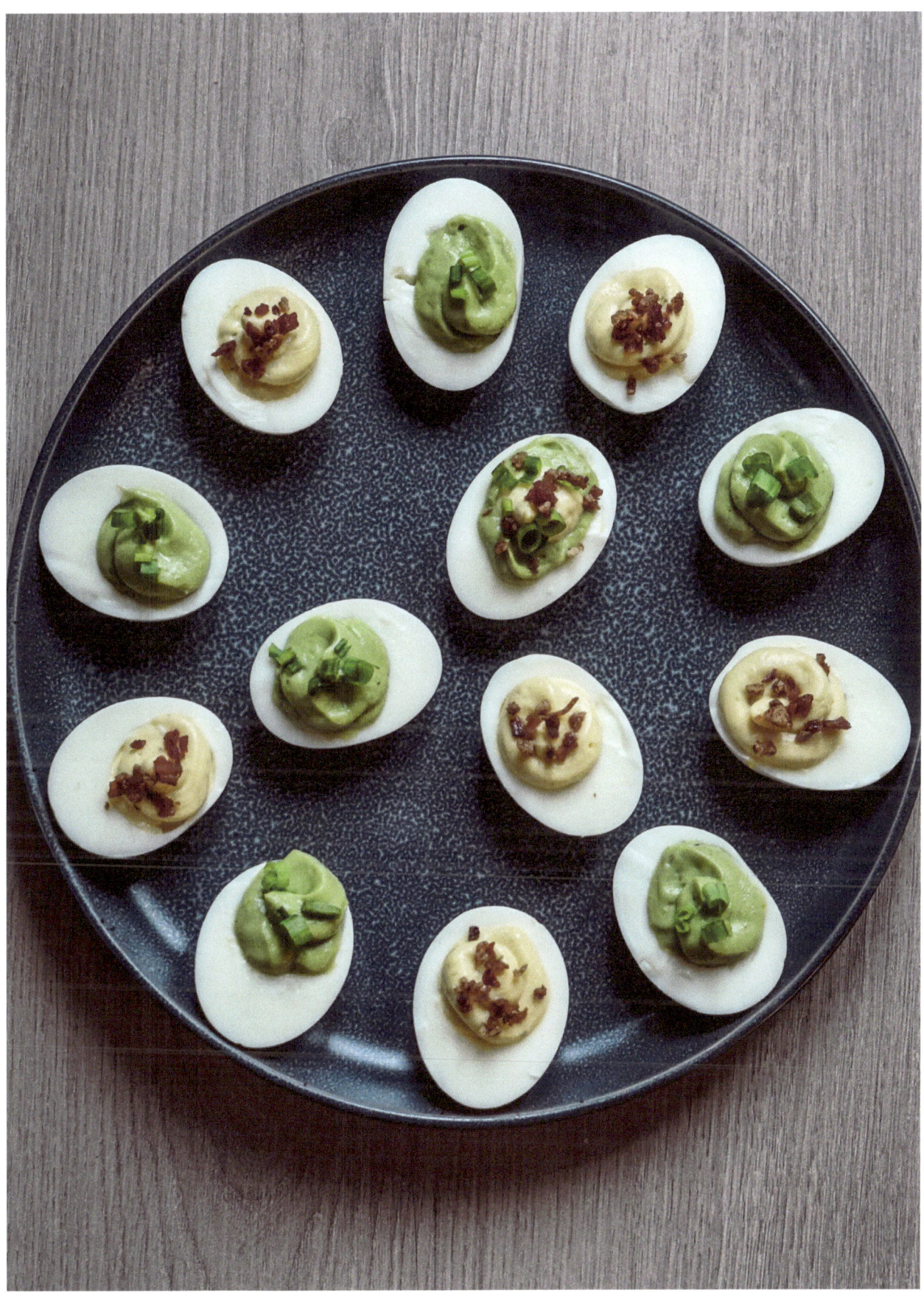

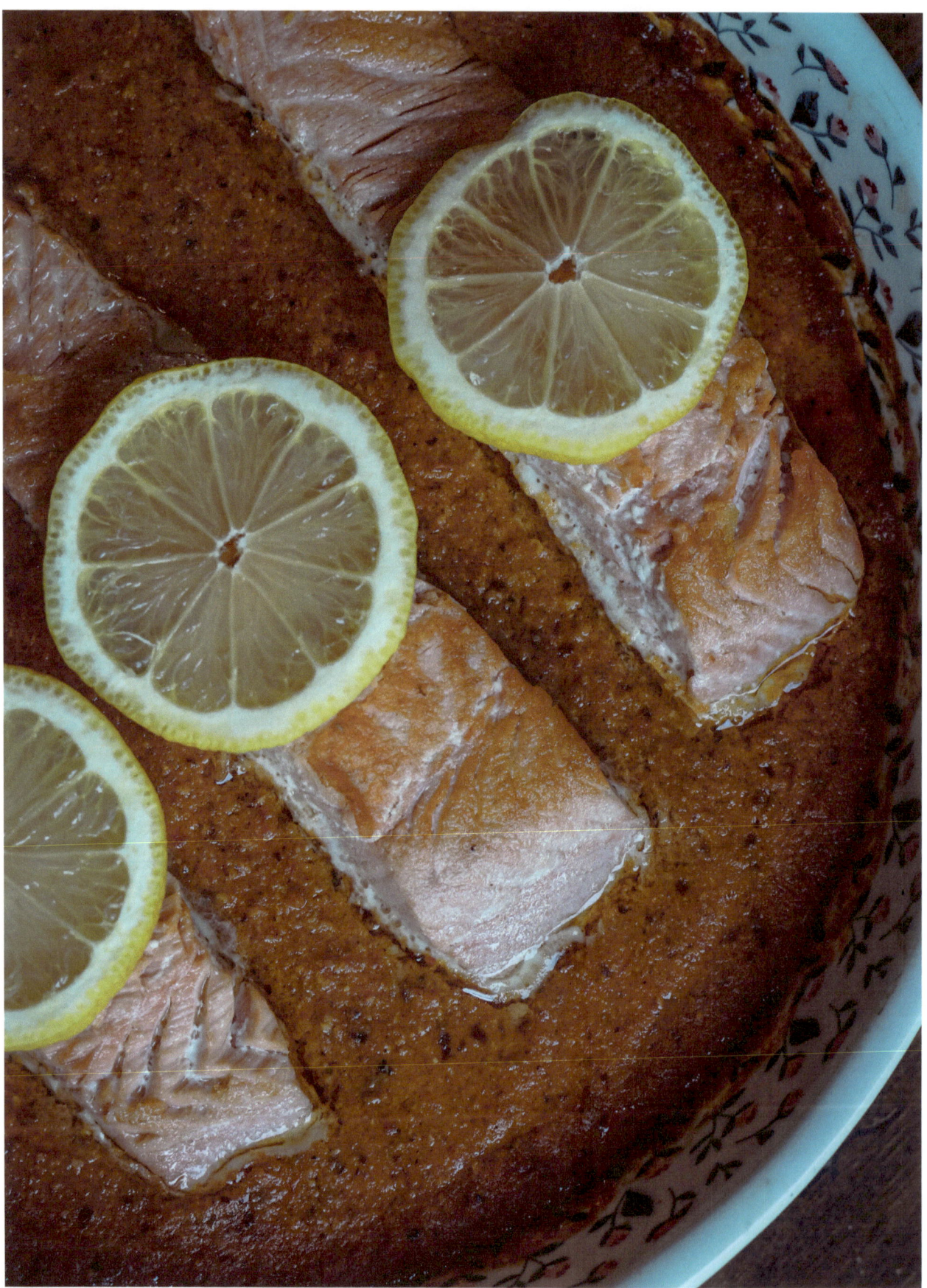

FEELING FLIRTY

ROASTED RED PEPPER SALMON

MAKES 4 SALMON
FILLETS + SAUCE

PAIRS WELL WITH:
- CANDLELIGHT
- MEDITERRANEAN PLAYLISTS
- LICKING THE PLATE

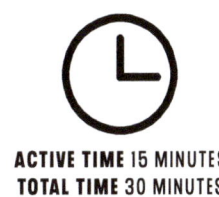

ACTIVE TIME 15 MINUTES
TOTAL TIME 30 MINUTES

SPECIAL EQUIPMENT

Baking dish
Blender

INGREDIENTS

SAUCE

1 cup roasted red pepper
½ cup smoked almonds
2 tomatoes, chopped
3 cloves garlic, diced
¼ cup red wine vinegar
2 teaspoons paprika
½ teaspoon red pepper flakes
½ cup coconut milk

SALMON

1 Tablespoon coconut, avocado or canola oil (something with a high smoke point)
4 salmon fillets, with the skin removed
8 lemon slices (2 per fillet)
2 Tablespoons fresh oregano
Salt and pepper to taste

SERVE WITH

Steamed veggies
Something to douse in sauce (rice or couscous are great)

INSTRUCTIONS

PREP THE SAUCE

Measure the red pepper, almonds, tomato, garlic, vinegar, paprika and red pepper flakes into a blender and mix until smooth.

Once blended, pour the mixture into a small saucepan, then stir in the coconut milk over low heat until warm. Cover and set aside - it's salmon time!

BATHE THE SALMON

Preheat the oven to 400°F.

Heat one tablespoon of oil in a large pan over medium heat.

Sear each salmon fillet until golden and crispy (about two minutes on each side). Depending on the size of the fillets, you may have to cook the salmon in two batches.

Pour the red pepper sauce into the oven-safe dish, place the salmon in the sauce, then add the lemon slices.

Bake for 10-15 minutes, until the salmon is no longer pink on the inside.

Remove from the oven, sprinkle with oregano, and serve!

Feeling Flirty

FRENCH SILK PIE

**MAKES 2 PIES
(ABOUT 16 SLICES)**

PAIRS WELL WITH:
- SILK PAJAMAS
- SHARING A SPOON
- LARGE GROUPS

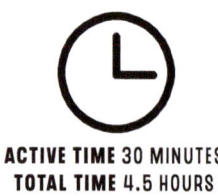

ACTIVE TIME 30 MINUTES
TOTAL TIME 4.5 HOURS

SPECIAL EQUIPMENT

Electric mixer, egg beater, or a well-caffeinated friend with a fork

INGREDIENTS

THE PIE

2 pre-made pie crusts
4 large eggs
1 ⅓ cups sugar
8 ounces bittersweet or semi-sweet chocolate, melted
2 teaspoons vanilla extract
10 Tablespoons butter/margarine, room temperature
1 ⅓ cups heavy cream or coconut cream
4 teaspoons powdered sugar

THE TOPPING

1 cup heavy cream or coconut cream
2 Tablespoons powdered sugar
1 teaspoon vanilla extract
Chocolate shavings or curls

HERE'S THE DEAL

Our recommendation is to make this pie the day before you want to eat it.

INSTRUCTIONS

Bake the pie crusts per the package instructions and set aside to cool.

MAKE THE BASE
Combine the eggs and sugar in a saucepan over medium-low heat. Whisk continuously until the temperature hits 160°F, then remove from heat.

Stir in the melted chocolate and vanilla until you have a smooth consistency, then set aside to cool.

WHISKY BUSINESS
Put the butter into a medium bowl and beat with an electric mixer until fluffy. Switch to the whisk attachment, then slowly add in the chocolate mixture, increasing the mixer speed to high until everything is fluffy (about five minutes).

In a separate bowl with clean beaters, mix the cream until it gets thicker and borderline fluffy (seeing a theme are we?). Mix in the powdered sugar until peaks start to form.

Working carefully not to smoosh the fluffiness, gently fold the cream into the chocolate mix with a spatula, then distribute the mixture evenly between both pie crusts.

Chill the pies in the fridge for two to four hours.

TOP IT OFF
Measure the cream, powdered sugar, and vanilla into a mixing bowl and beat on high until peaks form.

Pull the pies out of the fridge, cover the filling with the freshly whipped cream, and shave a bar of chocolate onto the top using a sharp knife or cheese grater.

Ta da! You just made fancy pie. Now go eat it cause it's freaking delicious.

HOT TIP
Letting the chocolate mixture cool to room temperature is VERY important. If you rush it, you may end up with more of a fudgy consistency than the light and fluffy one we're going for.

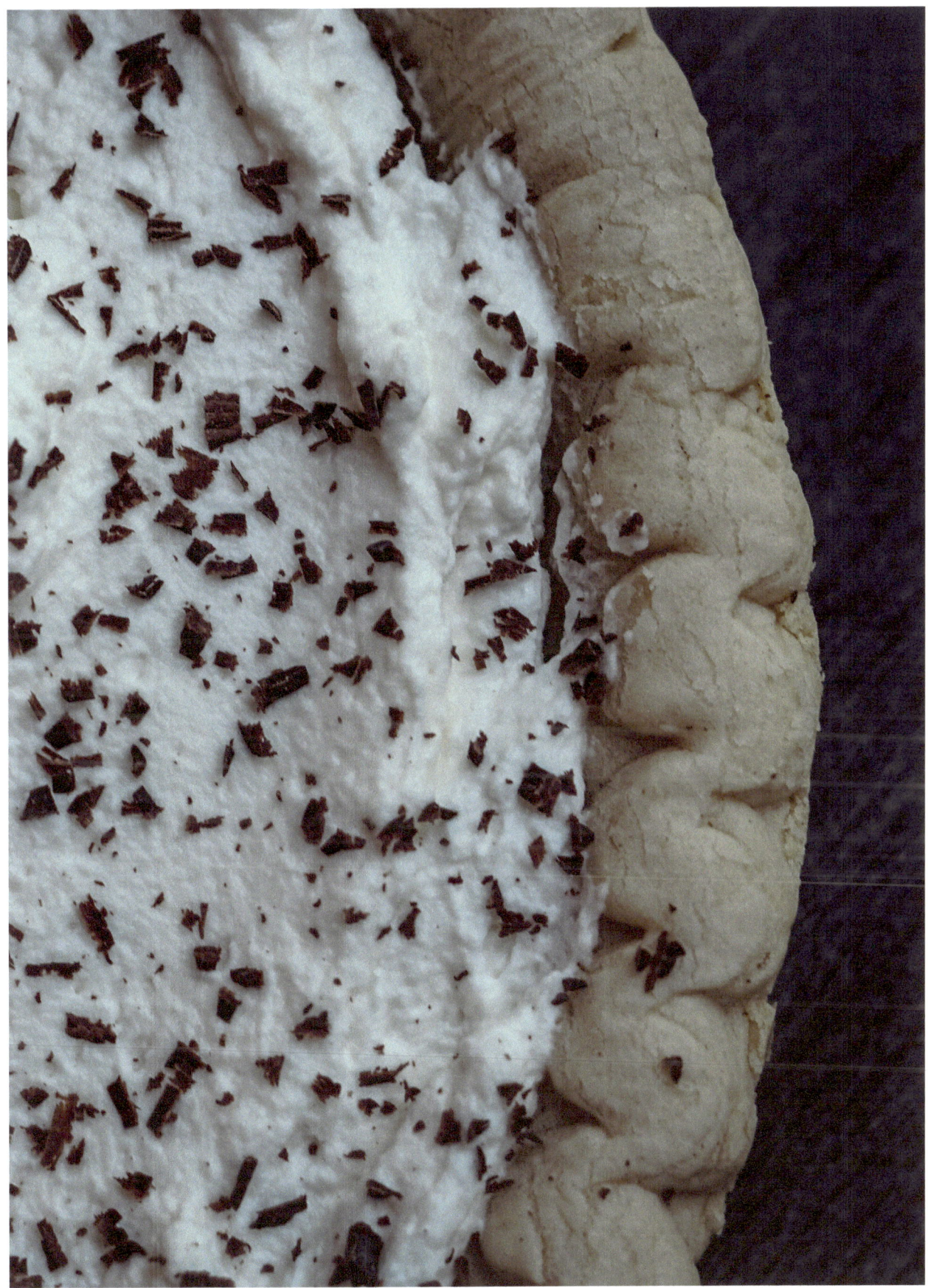

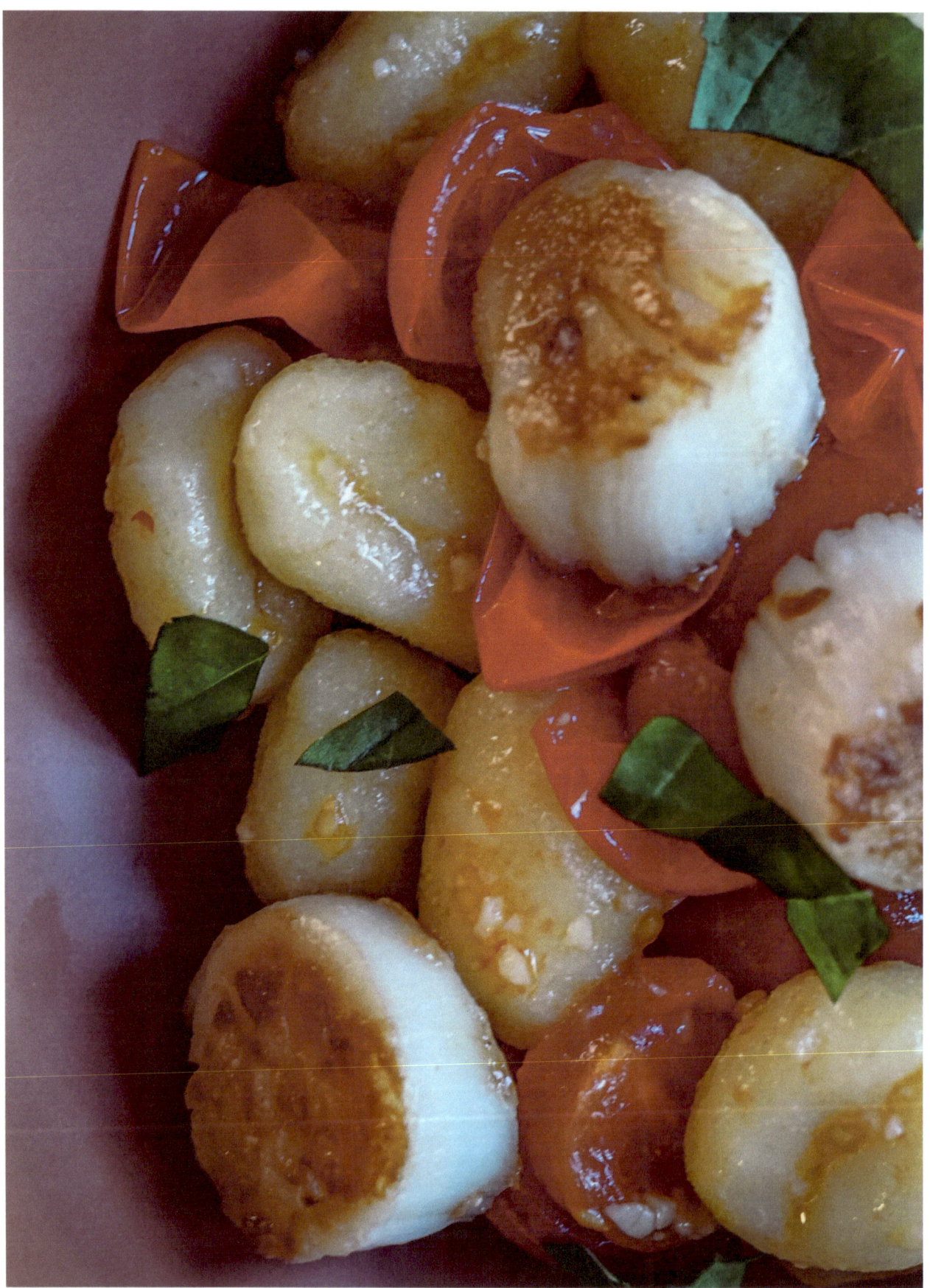

FEELING FLIRTY

SEARED SCALLOPS + GNOCCHI

MAKES 2 BOWLS

PAIRS WELL WITH:
- FANCY FORKS
- AGGRESSIVE CUDDLES
- SATISFACTION

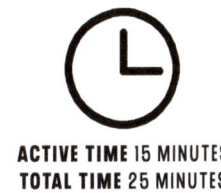

ACTIVE TIME 15 MINUTES
TOTAL TIME 25 MINUTES

INGREDIENTS

1 package gnocchi (18 ounces)
12 large scallops
1 Tablespoon coarse sea salt
1-2 Tablespoons avocado or other high-heat oil
2 cloves garlic, chopped
¼ cup olive oil or butter
1 pint cherry tomatoes, cut in half
1 Tablespoon sugar
¼ cup fresh basil, cut or torn
Parmesan cheese, for garnish (optional)

INSTRUCTIONS

Start by following the box directions to cook the gnocchi, then set it aside while you work on the scallops.

If you're starting with frozen scallops, be sure to thaw them out first by placing them in a cold water bath for an hour or until completely thawed. If using fresh scallops, proceed to the next step.

Place the scallops on a paper towel, pat dry then sprinkle sea salt on each side.

Heat a fry pan over high heat, then add the avocado oil.

When the oil is hot, add the scallops to the pan, being sure to keep a little space in between them. Depending on the size of your pan, you may have to cook the scallops in batches to prevent overcrowding.

Sear the scallops until golden and crispy (about 90 seconds on each side).

Remove the scallops from the pan and turn the stove down to medium heat.

Add the garlic and olive oil (or butter) to the pan, then sauté until the garlic is fragrant, about two or three minutes.

Toss in the tomatoes and sugar, and cook until they become soft and start to break down, about five minutes. The liquid should also now be thickening and becoming a light sauce so be sure to be stirring occasionally.

Pour the cooked gnocchi into the pan, use a spatula or wooden spoon to evenly coat it into the tomato sauce, then it's time to plate!

Create a bed of gnocchi-tomato-goodness in a shallow bowl or plate, top with an appropriate (or inappropriate) number of scallops, and garnish with basil and a light grating of parmesan.

Serve with a nice white wine.

Feeling Flirty

SMOKESHOW SALMON BENEDICT

MAKES 2 PLATES

PAIRS WELL WITH:
- USING SHEETS AS NAPKINS
- BREAKFAST IN BED
- THE CATCH OF THE DAY...
  OR THE NIGHT

TOTAL TIME 20 MINUTES

SPECIAL EQUIPMENT

Blender or immersion blender

INGREDIENTS

THE BASE
4 eggs
1 Tablespoon white vinegar
3 ounces smoked salmon
2 english muffins

THE HOLLANDAISE SAUCE
3 egg yolks
¼ teaspoon salt
¼ teaspoon pepper
1 Tablespoon lemon juice
½ cup unsalted butter, melted
2 teaspoons dill, chopped

HOT TIP

Want to make traditional eggs benedict instead? Swap the salmon for ham, add a slice of tomato, and remove the dill from the hollandaise in exchange for a pinch of cayenne.

INSTRUCTIONS

POACH THE EGGS

Start by bringing a small pot of water to a boil.

Crack each egg individually into a fine mesh sieve to strain the watery part of the egg off, then place it into a small bowl. If you don't have a sieve, leave your eggs in their shells and proceed to the next step.

Pour the tablespoon of vinegar into the boiling water, then swirl the water with a large spoon to create a little whirlpool.

While the whirlpool is still spinning, gently pour one egg from the small bowl into the center of the pot. If you didn't strain the eggs earlier, you can just crack each one directly into the water.
Each should be perfectly poached in about three minutes. Remove the egg with a slotted spoon and set aside, then repeat the whirlpool process until all the eggs are cooked.

MAKE THE HOLLANDAISE

Toss the egg yolks, salt, pepper, and lemon juice into the blender.

Start blending the egg mixture on high, then carefully open the lid and slowly pour the melted butter inside. Depending on the size of your blender lid and how lucky you feel, you could use a kitchen towel to cover some of the opening as you pour the butter in.

Once the majority of the butter is in the blender, the sauce should be thick. Sample the sauce and feel free to add lemon juice, salt, or pepper to suit your taste buds, then stir in the dill and taste it again.

PLATE IT UP

Toast the english muffins, place a few slices of smoked salmon on each one, then add a poached egg on top. Douse the stack in hollandaise, sprinkle with a little dill, and enjoy!

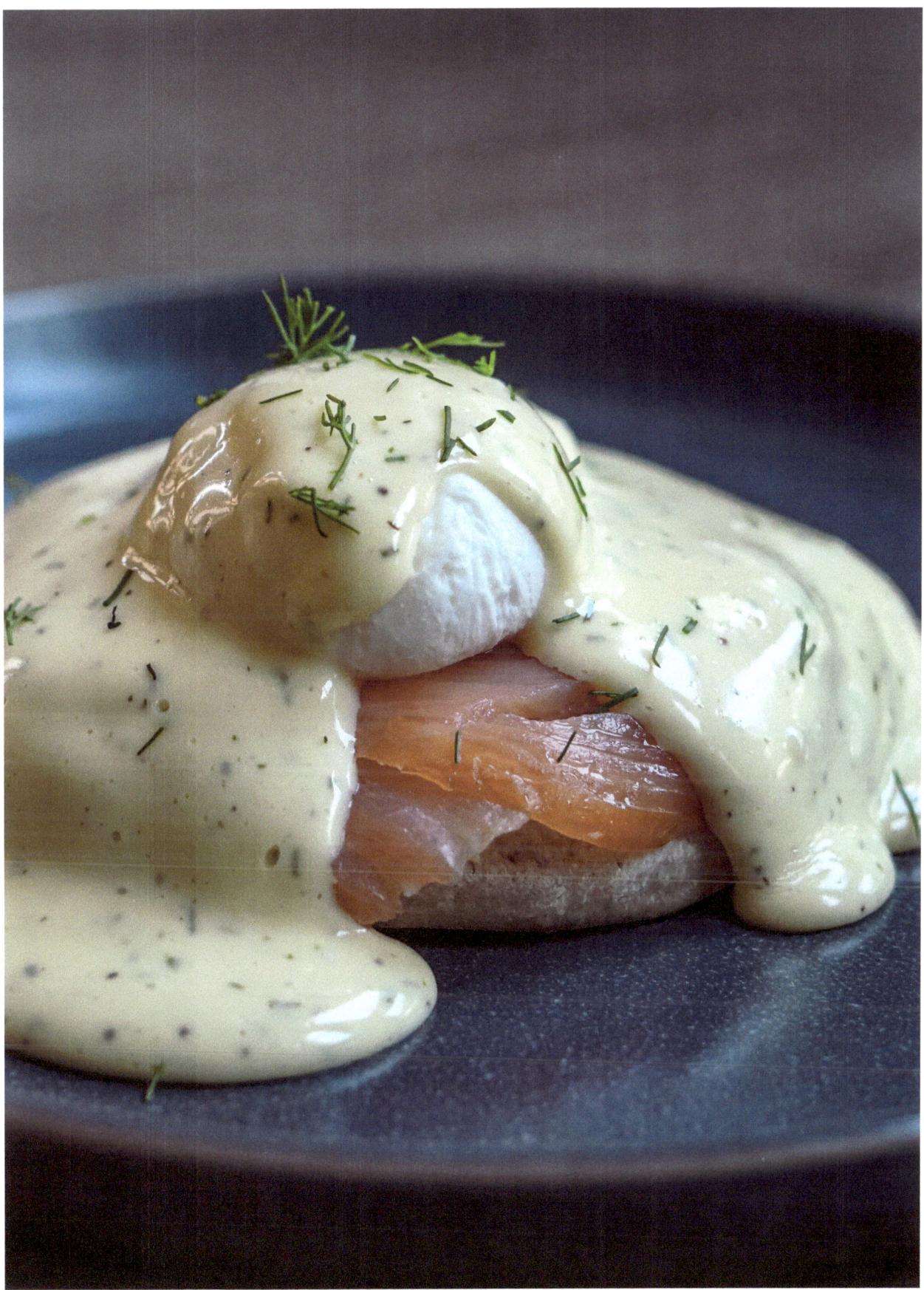

FEELING FLIRTY

NEW YORK SOUR

MAKES 1 DRINK

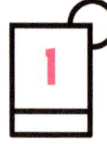

PAIRS WELL WITH:
- WELL-DRESSED DATES
- WANTING IT ALL
- MATCHING YOUR DRINK TO YOUR LIPSTICK

TOTAL TIME
2 MINUTES

SPECIAL EQUIPMENT
Cocktail shaker
Rocks glass (optional)

INGREDIENTS
- 2 ounces rye or bourbon whiskey
- 1 ounce lemon juice
- 1 ounce simple syrup
- ½ ounce dry or fruity red wine (whatever you're feeling)

INSTRUCTIONS
- Combine whiskey, lemon juice and simple syrup in a cocktail shaker full of ice.
- Cover and shake until chilled (about 30 seconds).
- Strain into a rocks glass filled with ice.
- To finish, pour the wine over the back of a spoon into the glass - the spoon will help the wine float on top of the drink, which looks pretty cool, if you ask us. Ta-Done!

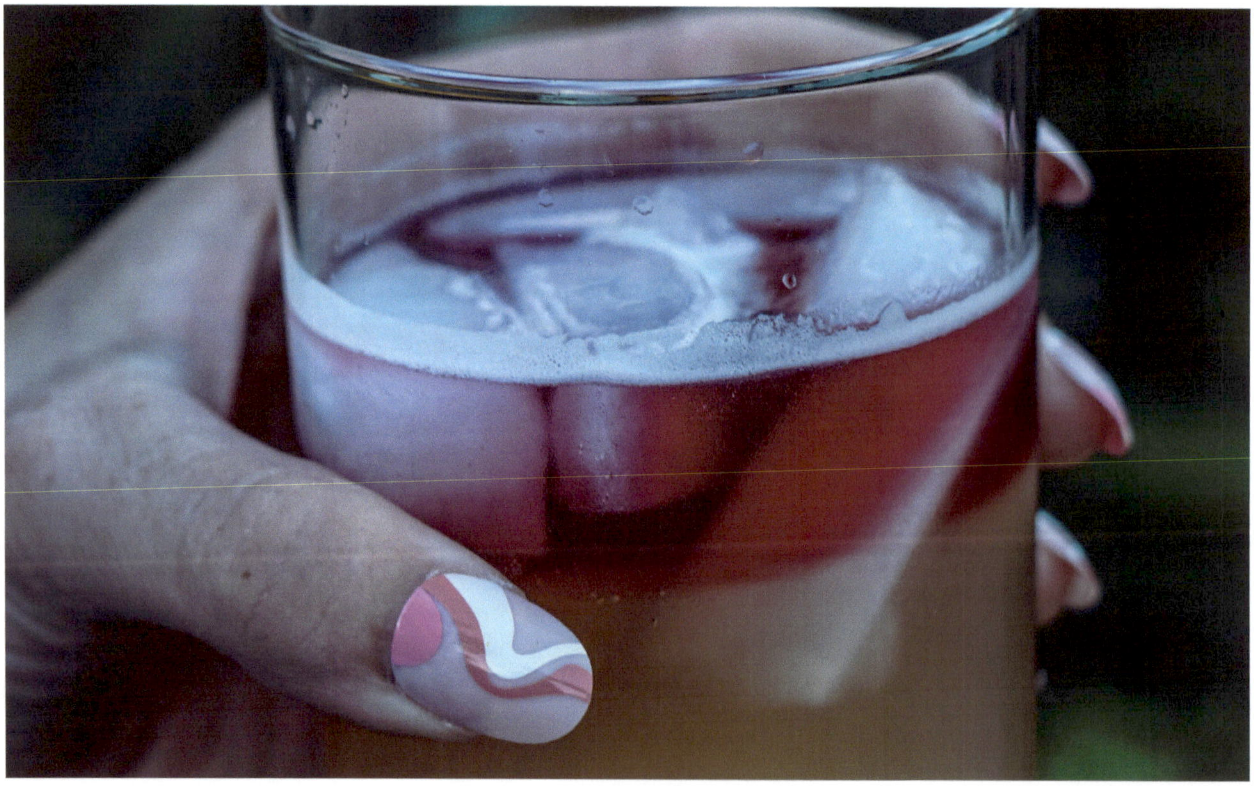

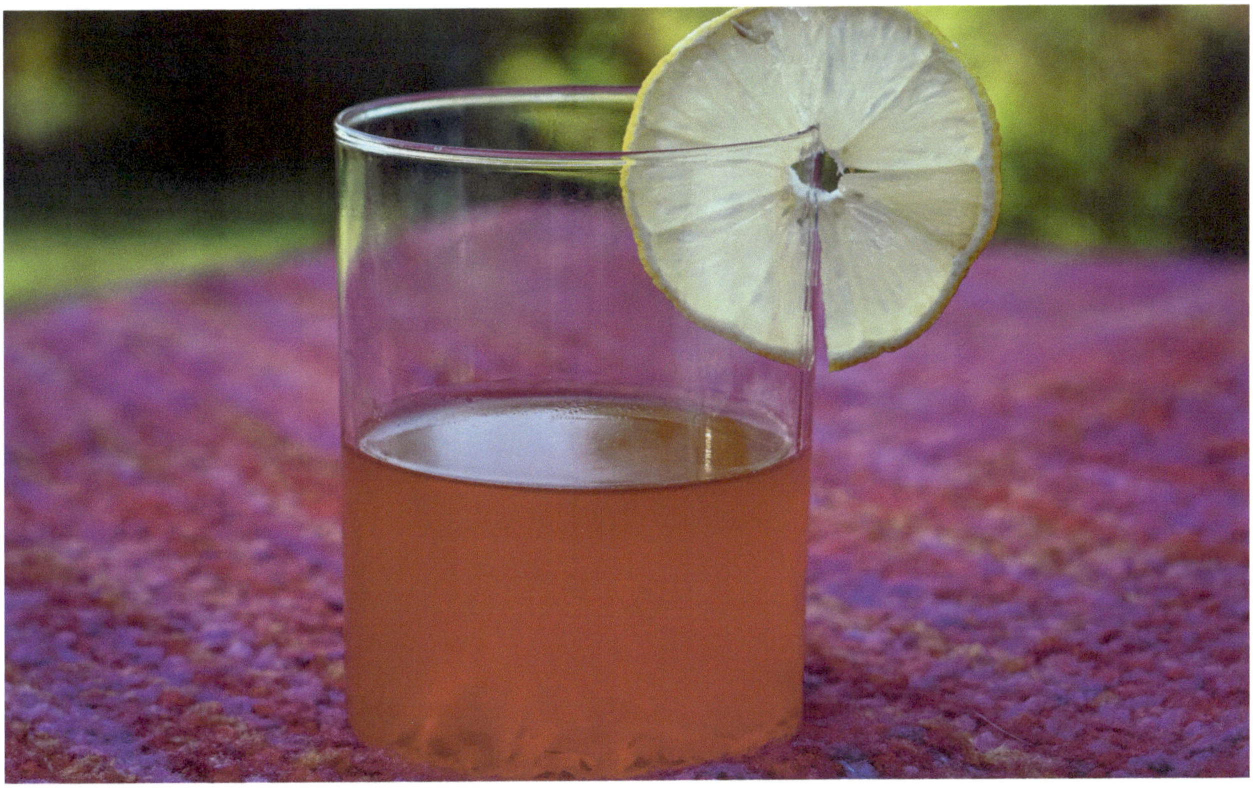

PAPER PLANES

MAKES 1 DRINK

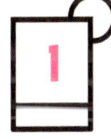

PAIRS WELL WITH:
- VELVET. ALL THE VELVET.
- HAWAIIAN PUNCH CRAVINGS
- BIG GIRL PANTS

TOTAL TIME
2 MINUTES

INGREDIENTS
- 1 ounce bourbon
- 1 ounce aperol
- 1 ounce italian amaro
- 1 ounce fresh-squeezed lemon juice
- Lemon peel for garnish
- Fresh ice

INSTRUCTIONS
- Pour equal parts bourbon, aperol, amaro, and lemon juice into a cocktail shaker.
- Fill the rest of the shaker with ice and shake until everything is cold (about 30 seconds).
- Strain into a cocktail glass and garnish with lemon peel or pink fruit for a little more sweetness.

FEELING

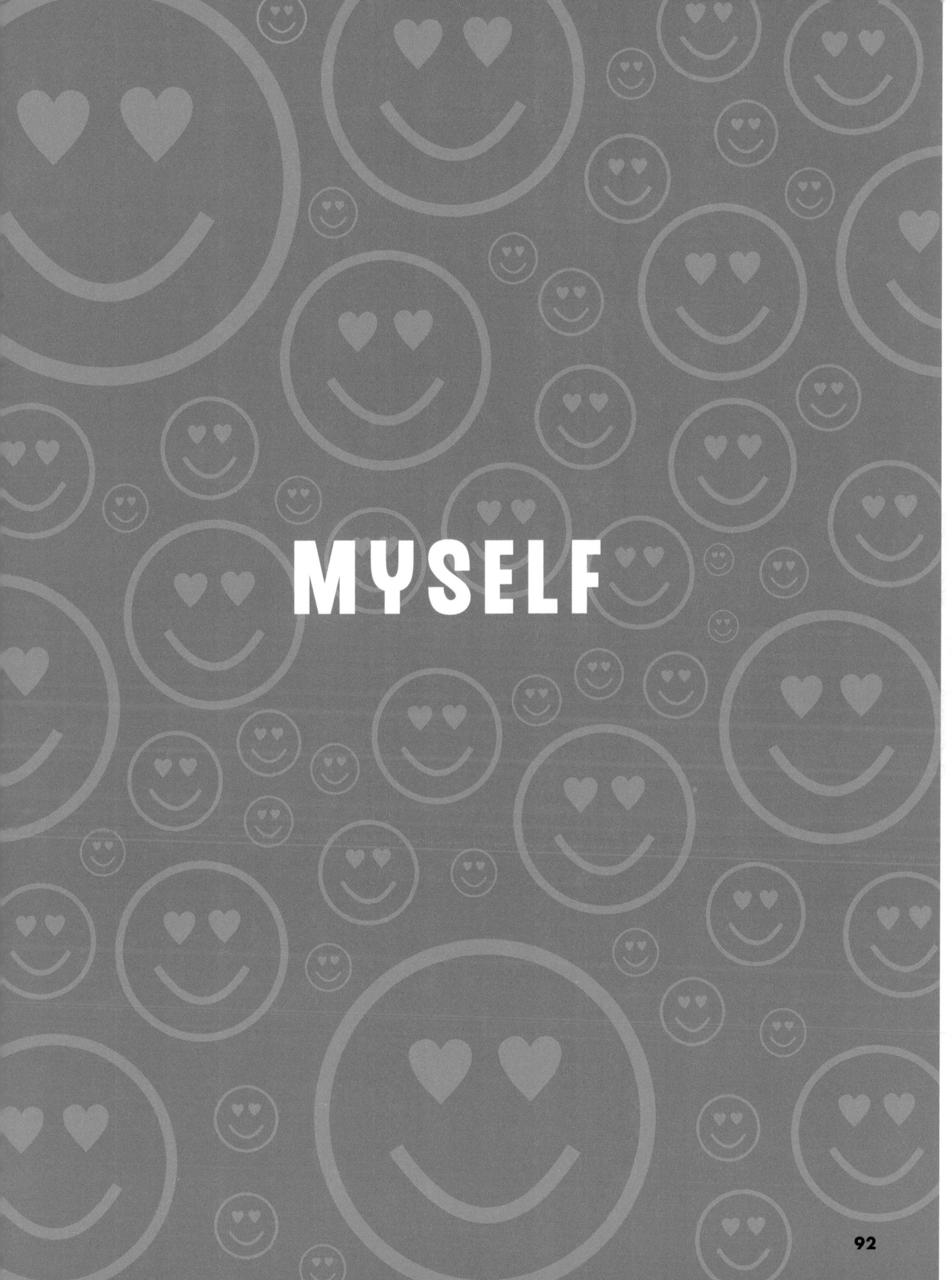

FEELING MYSELF

SASSY SHRIMP TACOS

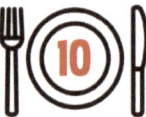

MAKES 10 TACOS

PAIRS WELL WITH:
• FEEDING YOURSELF FOR THE WEEK
• PINEAPPLE MARGARITAS
• HEALTH KICKS

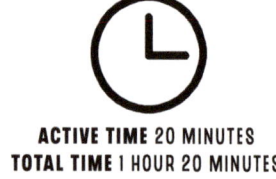

ACTIVE TIME 20 MINUTES
TOTAL TIME 1 HOUR 20 MINUTES

SPECIAL EQUIPMENT

Cast iron pan
Food processor or blender

INGREDIENTS

MARINADE
1 pound frozen cooked shrimp, thawed and tails removed
1 teaspoon chili powder
1 teaspoon smoked paprika
1 teaspoon minced garlic
1 teaspoon red pepper flakes
½ teaspoon ground cumin
½ teaspoon dried oregano
½ teaspoon salt
1 lime, juiced
3 Tablespoon olive oil

AVOCADO CREAM
1 large avocado
½ cup cilantro
1 jalapeno, seeds removed
3 cloves garlic
2 limes, juiced
½ cup plain greek yogurt
3 Tablespoons olive oil
3 Tablespoons water
½ teaspoon kosher salt

TACOS
1 cup green cabbage, shredded
1 cup purple cabbage, shredded
10 taco-sized tortillas (corn or flour)
Chilis in Adobo (optional, see note to the right)
Fresh cilantro
Lime wedges

INSTRUCTIONS

In a small bowl whisk together the marinade ingredients, then toss in the shrimp.

Place the mixture in the refrigerator to chill for at least an hour.

While the shrimp marinades, measure the avocado cream ingredients into a food processor and pulse until smooth.

Shred the cabbage.

Heat a cast iron pan on medium-high heat, then remove the shrimp from the fridge and add it to the pan. Cook for two minutes, flipping halfway through, then remove the shrimp from the pan so you can use it to heat up the tortillas!

Place a pinch of cabbage at the bottom of each tortilla, add shrimp, and drizzle with avocado cream.

Top with cilantro and lime and enjoy!

FEELING COLORFUL?

Add a bit of spice (and color) to your tacos. Blend ½ cup water with a 7-ounce can of Chilies in Adobo until smooth, then pour into a large mixing bowl or shallow pan. Dip one tortilla at a time into the mixture, then cook each side over medium-low heat.

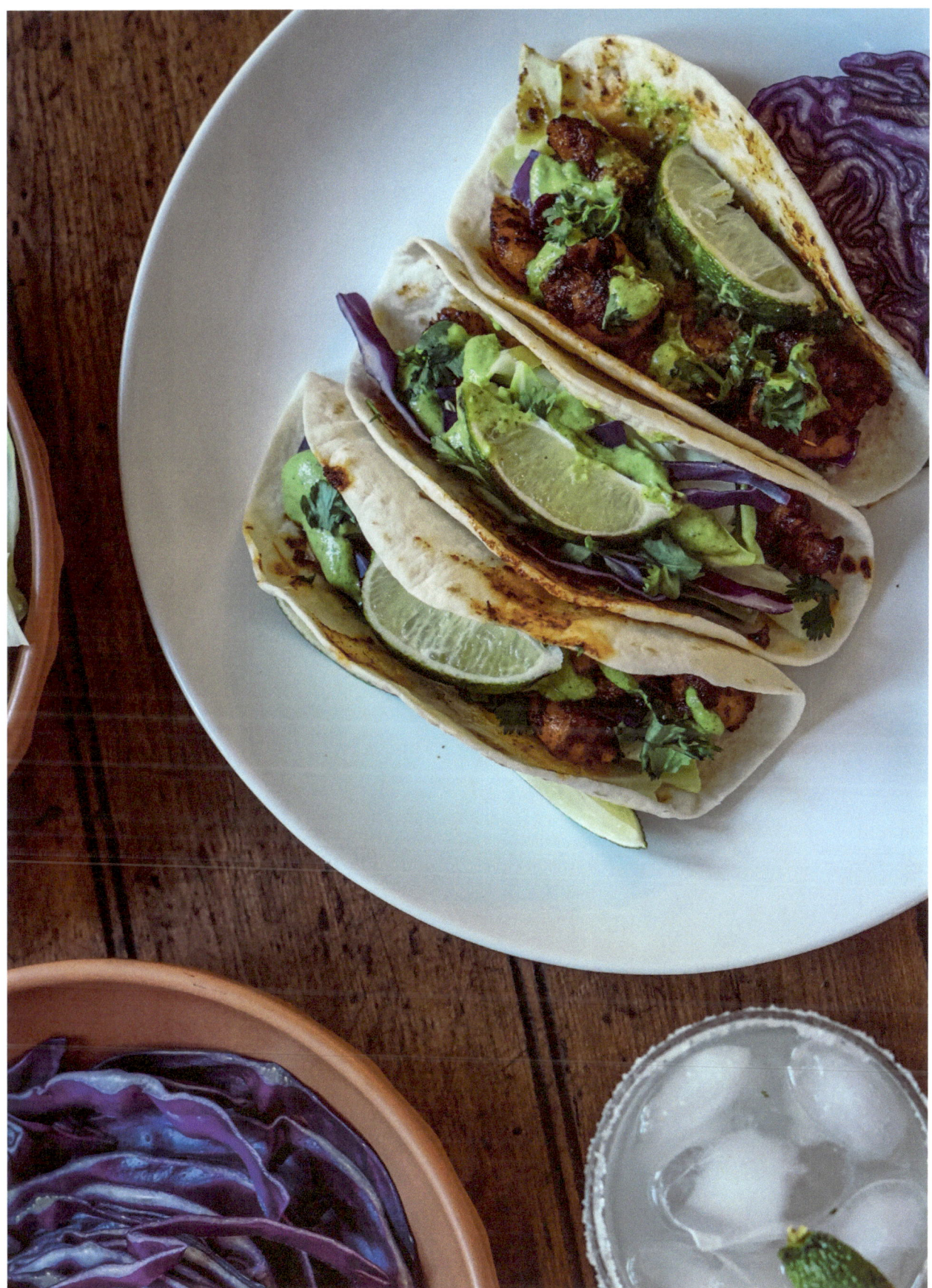

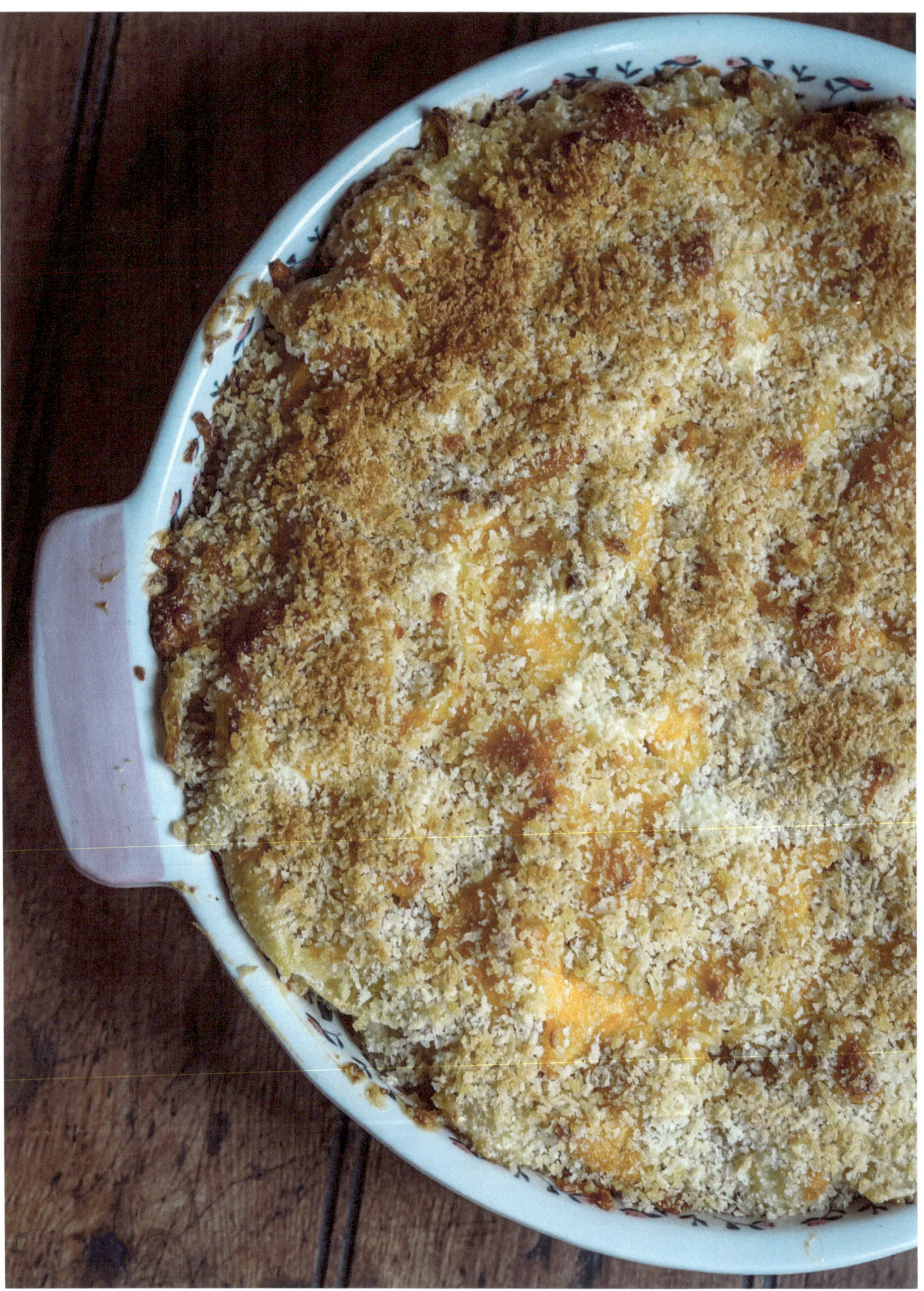

GF

FEELING MYSELF

BAKED MAC AND CHEESE

MAKES 6 SERVINGS
(3 IF YOU'RE HANGRY)

PAIRS WELL WITH:
- AFFIRMATIONS
- GOOD FRIENDS
- CHEAP WINE

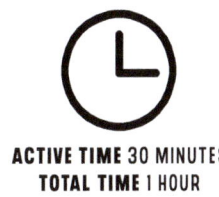

ACTIVE TIME 30 MINUTES
TOTAL TIME 1 HOUR

SPECIAL EQUIPMENT

Whisk
9x13 glass baking pan

INGREDIENTS

2 cups medium shell noodles
1 cup cheddar cheese, grated
1 cup grated gruyere cheese
1 cup grated swiss cheese
½ cup additional grated cheese for topping
3 Tablespoons butter
¼ cup flour
2 cups heavy cream
¼ teaspoon salt
¼ teaspoon pepper
½ teaspoon paprika
1 ½ teaspoon dry mustard
1 cup panko bread crumbs
Hot sauce (optional)

CHEESY TIP

Pre-shredded cheese is coated to prevent it from sticking together in the bag. Unless you enjoy a really stringy texture, we recommend buying the cheese in blocks and grating it yourself.

INSTRUCTIONS

Cook the pasta al dente according to box instructions, then rinse with cold water and set aside.

Shred and mix the varieties of cheese together.

Melt the butter in a large saucepan or pot over medium heat. Slowly whisk in the flour until smooth (about three minutes).

Slowly whisk in one cup of the cream, doing your best to keep the mixture smooth.

After the cream is incorporated, add the salt, pepper, paprika, and dry mustard.

Stir for an additional 10-12 minutes or until the sauce has thickened.

Remove from heat and slowly mix in the three cups of shredded cheese, about a handful at a time until it has all melted and looks like a delicious sauce.

Toss in the noodles and stir to evenly coat them with cheesy goodness.

Pour the cheesy mixture into a 9x13 glass baking pan. Toss on the cheese you set aside at the beginning for the top and sprinkle with the breadcrumbs.

Bake until lightly golden brown (about 30 minutes on the middle rack), then set your oven to broil! This will give the breadcrumbs a rich golden brown, but be sure to keep an eye on the pan to ensure it doesn't burn.

Remove the mac from the oven. Drizzle with hot sauce if you're so inclined or serve it up as-is and enjoy!

FEELING MYSELF

SEA SALT + CHOCOLATE CHIP COOKIES

MAKES 18 COOKIES

PAIRS WELL WITH:
- NEW SHOES
- MONDAYS
- ANY OF THE MILKS

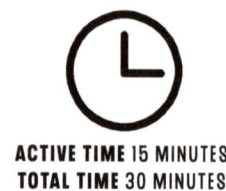

ACTIVE TIME 15 MINUTES
TOTAL TIME 30 MINUTES

SPECIAL EQUIPMENT

2 baking sheets

INGREDIENTS

¾ cup brown sugar, packed
½ cup granulated sugar
4 Tablespoons butter, softened
¼ cup olive oil (yes, olive oil!)
1 egg
1 teaspoon vanilla
1 ½ cups flour
½ teaspoon baking soda
½ teaspoon baking powder
½ teaspoon salt
8 ounces chocolate chips, any variety
Sea salt for garnish

INSTRUCTIONS

MAKE THE DOUGH

Mix together the brown sugar, granulated sugar, butter, and olive oil in a large bowl.

Add the egg and vanilla and continue mixing until well combined.

In another large bowl, combine the flour, baking soda, baking powder, and salt. Mix thoroughly.

Stir the dry mix into the wet mix until they form one homogenous dough, then add the chocolate chips.

At this point you can go ahead and bake the dough, or you can stick it in the refrigerator and save it for later. Putting it in the fridge overnight will age the dough and richen the color and flavors.

BAKE THE DOUGH

Preheat your oven to 350°F, and line a couple of baking sheets with parchment paper.

Pick up a small amount of dough, roll into a ball with your hands, and place onto the baking sheet.

Rinse and repeat! You should be able to fit about nine cookies on each sheet.

Bake until the cookies are golden brown (about 10-13 minutes), or you start pacing near the oven.

Remove from the oven, sprinkle with sea salt, then let the cookies rest for a few minutes. Once rested, they can be moved to a cooling rack.

Nom to your heart's content, then share with your friends. Or not. It's your kitchen!

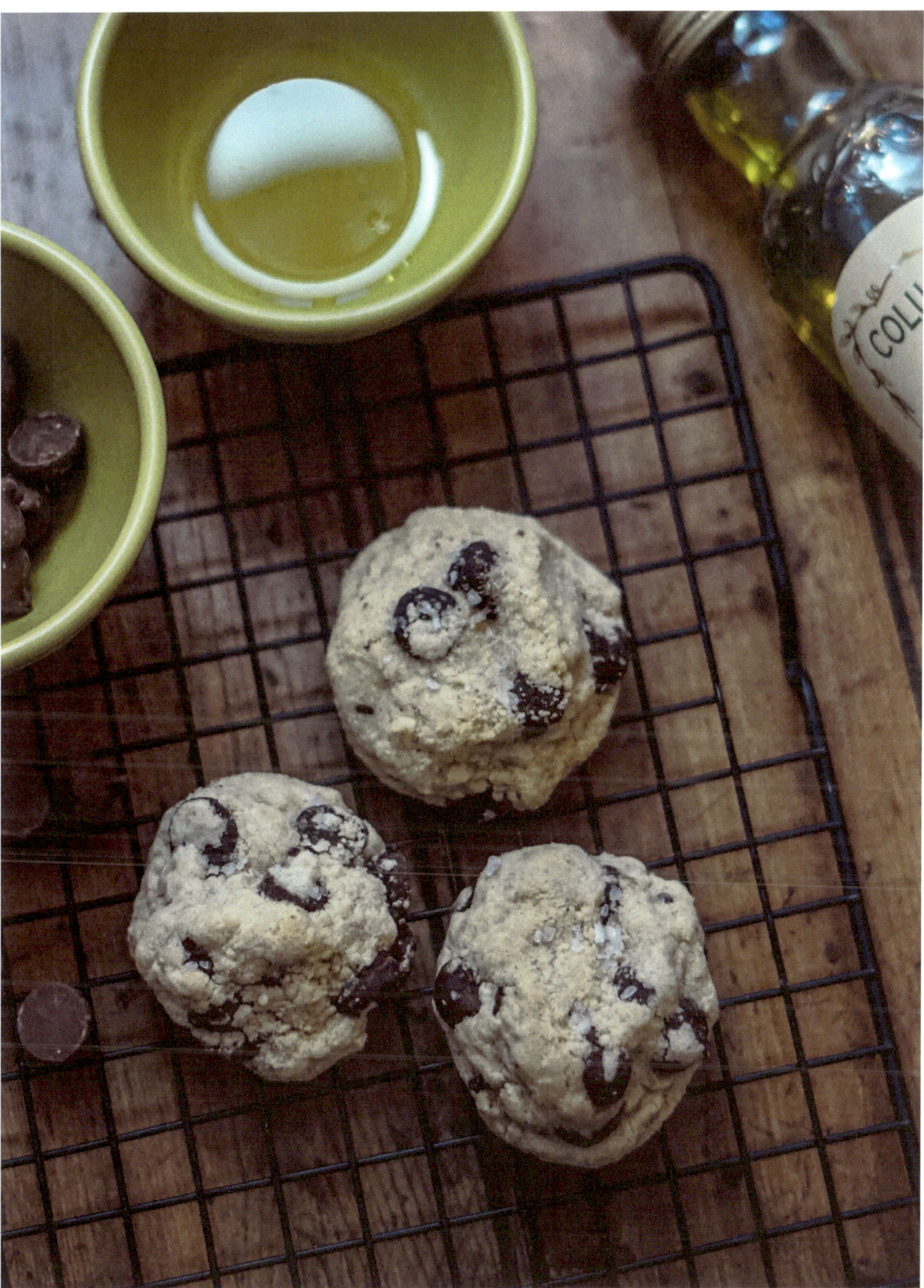

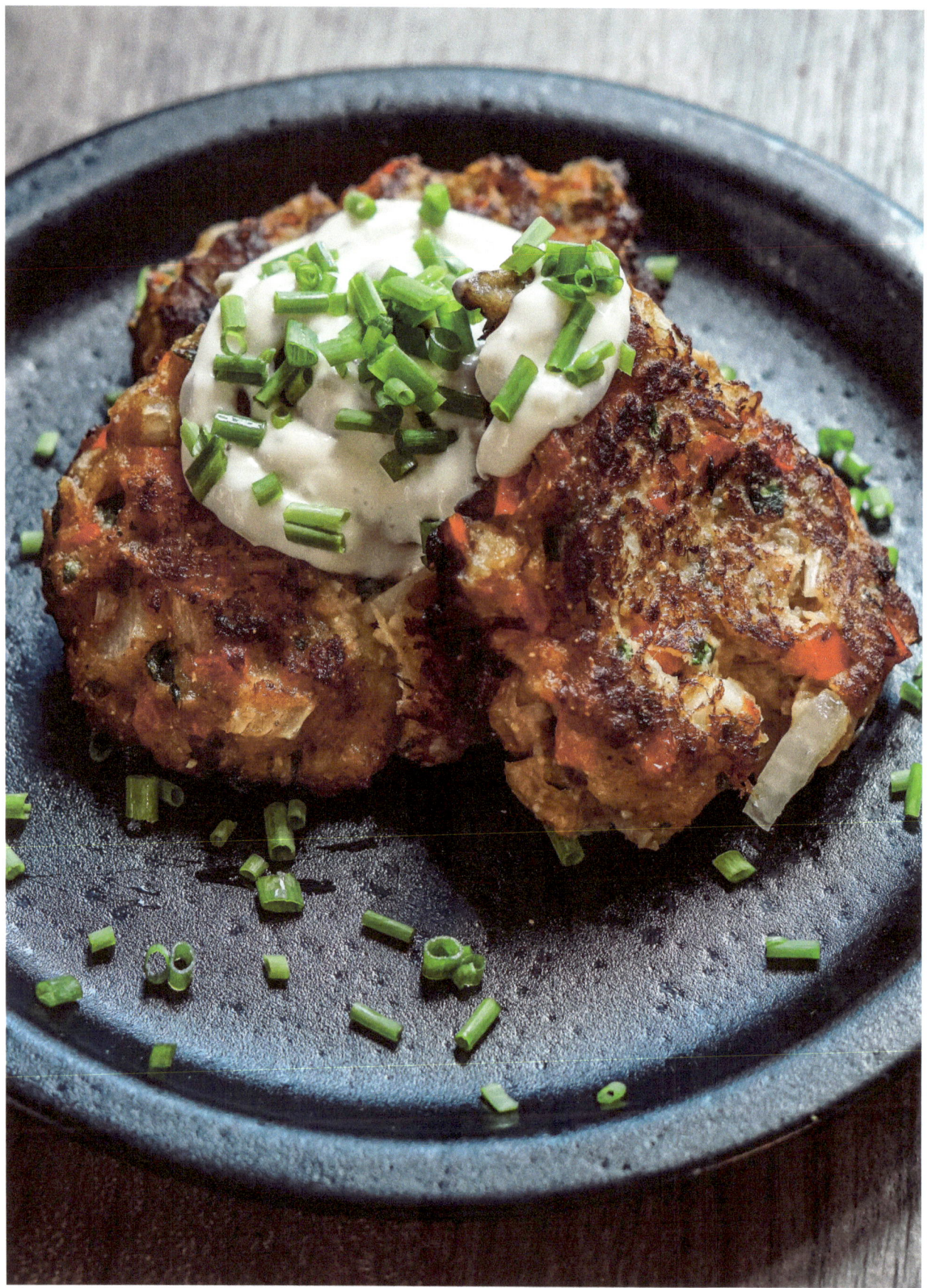

FEELING MYSELF

SALMON CROQUETTES

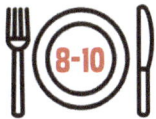

MAKES 8-10 CROQUETTES

PAIRS WELL WITH:
- WANDERLUST
- LEFTOVER SALMON
- LOTS OF LEMONS

TOTAL TIME 30 MINUTES

SPECIAL EQUIPMENT

Large pot
Meat or candy thermometer

INGREDIENTS

¼ cup flour
½ cup panko bread crumbs
15 ounces canned salmon
1 bell pepper, diced
¾ cup yellow onion, diced
1 egg, beaten
1 Tablespoon worcestershire sauce
1 teaspoon salt
½ teaspoon pepper
1 teaspoon garlic powder
¼ cup mayo
¼ cup cilantro, chopped
1-2 cups canola or vegetable oil, for frying
Lemon wedges and tartar sauce, for garnish

INSTRUCTIONS

Start by whisking together the flour and bread crumbs in a large bowl.

Add the rest of the ingredients (except the oil, lemon, and tartar sauce of course) to the bowl and stir.

Lay a sheet of parchment paper (about the size of a baking sheet) on the counter.

Take a handful of the salmon mix, shape it into a pattie, and place it on the parchment.

Repeat until the mix is gone. You should get 8-10 patties, depending on the size of your hands, of course.

Fill a deep-sided pan with ½" of oil over medium-high heat.

Once the oil is hot (350°F-375°F), gently place a few patties into the pan, being careful not to splash hot oil on yourself!

Fry each pattie until golden brown (about three minutes per side), then remove and place on a plate lined with paper towels to cool.

Serve with tartar sauce, lemon wedges, and a smile. :)

FEELING MYSELF

CRUNKWRAPS

MAKES 6 WRAPS

PAIRS WELL WITH:
• LATE NIGHT SODIUM NEEDS
• LEFTOVER TACO SAUCE PACKETS
• HEAPS OF SALSA

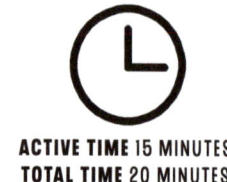

ACTIVE TIME 15 MINUTES
TOTAL TIME 20 MINUTES

SPECIAL EQUIPMENT

Griddle (handy but not necessary)

INGREDIENTS

1 pound ground beef (or plant-based alternative)
2+ cups shredded lettuce, any variety
1 tomato, diced
1 packet taco seasoning
1 jar salsa con queso (can substitute queso blanco)
6 of the biggest flour tortillas you can find
6 tostadas (flat, round, crunchy taco shells)
1 cup sour cream
1 cup shredded mexican cheese
Cooking spray

INSTRUCTIONS

PREP
Brown the beef over medium heat in a large pan. While the beef is cooking, chop and dice your lettuce and tomato.
Once the beef is browned, drain the fat into a disposable container, return beef to the pan and add the taco seasoning packet and water (following seasoning packet instructions).
Stir over heat until the moisture dissapates and the seasoning is well distributed. Set aside.
Heat the queso dip, being careful not to boil it.

LAYER UP
Lay the tortillas out onto a clean, flat surface, then layer the other ingredients into the center of each tortilla as follows:
One large spoonful of queso
⅓ cup scoop of beef
One tostada shell
A generous smear of sour cream
One small handful of lettuce
A sprinkle of tomato
A pinch of shredded cheese

TIME TO FOLD
Fold the outside of the tortilla in towards the middle, keeping the filling tightly wrapped without breaking the tortilla. You should end up with about six folds.

CRISP IT UP
Warm a griddle or a fry pan over medium heat and spray with cooking spray. Place one wrap onto the pan, folded side down, and cook until the tortilla is golden brown (about three minutes).
Use a large spatula to flip it over, brown the other side, then repeat until all the wraps are done.

Serve with taco sauce, guacamole and any leftover queso.

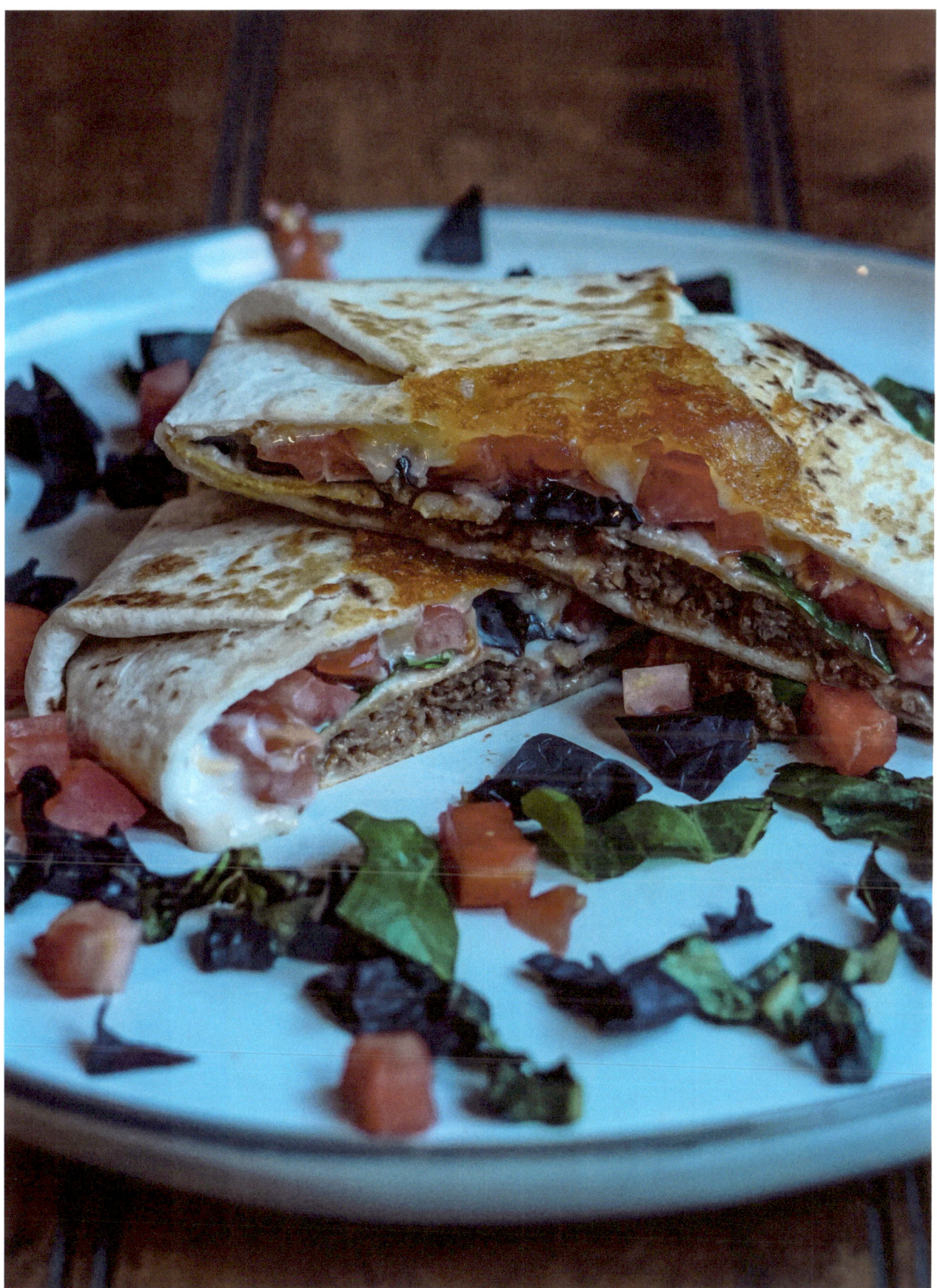

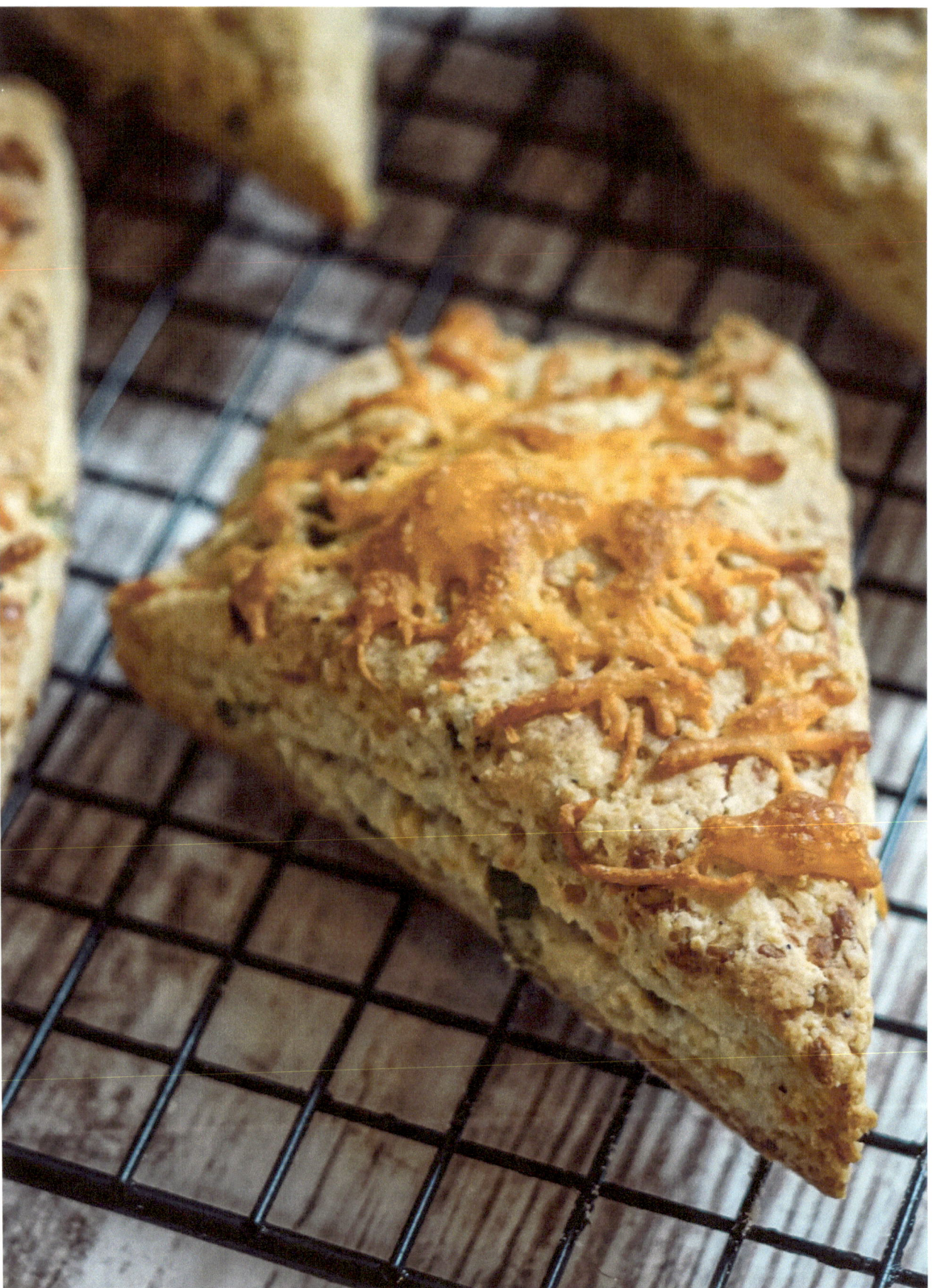

GF

FEELING MYSELF

CHEDDAR + SCALLION SCONES

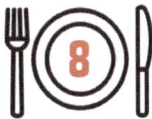

MAKES 8 SCONES

PAIRS WELL WITH:
- LATE STARTS
- READING THE ACTUAL NEWSPAPER
- A HOT CUP OF COFFEE

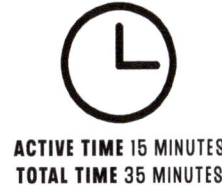

ACTIVE TIME 15 MINUTES
TOTAL TIME 35 MINUTES

SPECIAL EQUIPMENT

Baking sheet

INGREDIENTS

2 cups all purpose flour
½ Tablespoon sugar
½ teaspoon salt
2 teaspoons baking powder
½ teaspoon black pepper
5 Tablespoons butter, cut into cubes
½ cup cheddar cheese, shredded
4 scallions (A.K.A. green onions), sliced
½ cup milk or cream
2 eggs

INSTRUCTIONS

Preheat the oven to 400°F.

Stir together the flour, sugar, salt, baking powder, and black pepper.

Add the butter cubes to your dry mix and work them together with a fork or a pastry cutter until you create something resembling "peas" of flour butter, or crumbly sand.

Toss in the cheddar and scallions and stir until they are evenly distributed among the crumblies.

In another bowl, mix together the milk and eggs.

Pour this mixture into the bowl of crumblies and mix until a ball of dough forms.

Next, sprinkle flour onto a countertop to prevent the dough from sticking to it.

Remove the ball of dough from the bowl, use your hands to pack it into a tighter ball (as needed), then place it on the floured surface.

Press the ball into a one-inch thick circle (about the width of a dinner plate), then cut it into eight sections, like a pie.

Line a baking sheet with parchment paper, then carefully transfer each scone to the parchment, leaving a finger's width of room between each one.

Bake until golden brown (about 18-20 minutes), then eat while the cheese is nice and melty.

FEELING MYSELF

MARRY MYSELF CHICKEN

MAKES 4 PLATES

PAIRS WELL WITH:
- WELL-DESERVED RAISES
- BIG QUESTIONS
- LONG WEEKS

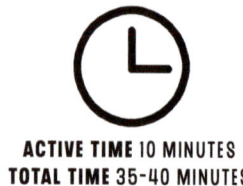

ACTIVE TIME 10 MINUTES
TOTAL TIME 35-40 MINUTES

SPECIAL EQUIPMENT

Blender
Meat thermometer

INGREDIENTS

1 Tablespoon olive oil
4 chicken breasts, fat trimmed away
Salt and pepper
3 cloves garlic, minced
1 teaspoon thyme (oregano will work)
Red pepper flakes, to taste (½ tsp = medium)
1 cup chicken broth
½ cup coconut cream (heavy cream works too)
½ cup chopped sun dried tomatoes
¼ cup grated parmesan (optional)
Fresh basil for garnish

INSTRUCTIONS

Preheat the oven to 375°F.

Heat the olive oil in a pan over medium-high heat.

Lightly season the chicken with salt and pepper, then gently place it into the pan.

Sear until golden brown (about four minutes per side), then pull the chicken out of the pan and set it aside.

Lower the heat to medium, add the garlic to the same (now empty) pan and cook until fragrant.

Toss in the thyme, red pepper flakes, broth and coconut cream, then stir and cook for five minutes.

Add the sundried tomatoes and parmesan cheese and stir again.

Pour the entire contents of the pan into a blender and blend on medium for 30-60 seconds, creating a rich, smooth sauce.

Place the chicken into an oven safe dish, then pour the sauce in and sprinkle with parmesan.

Bake for 25-30 minutes, until the chicken's internal temperature is 165°F.

Remove from the oven, plate, garnish with basil and additional parmesan, and enjoy!

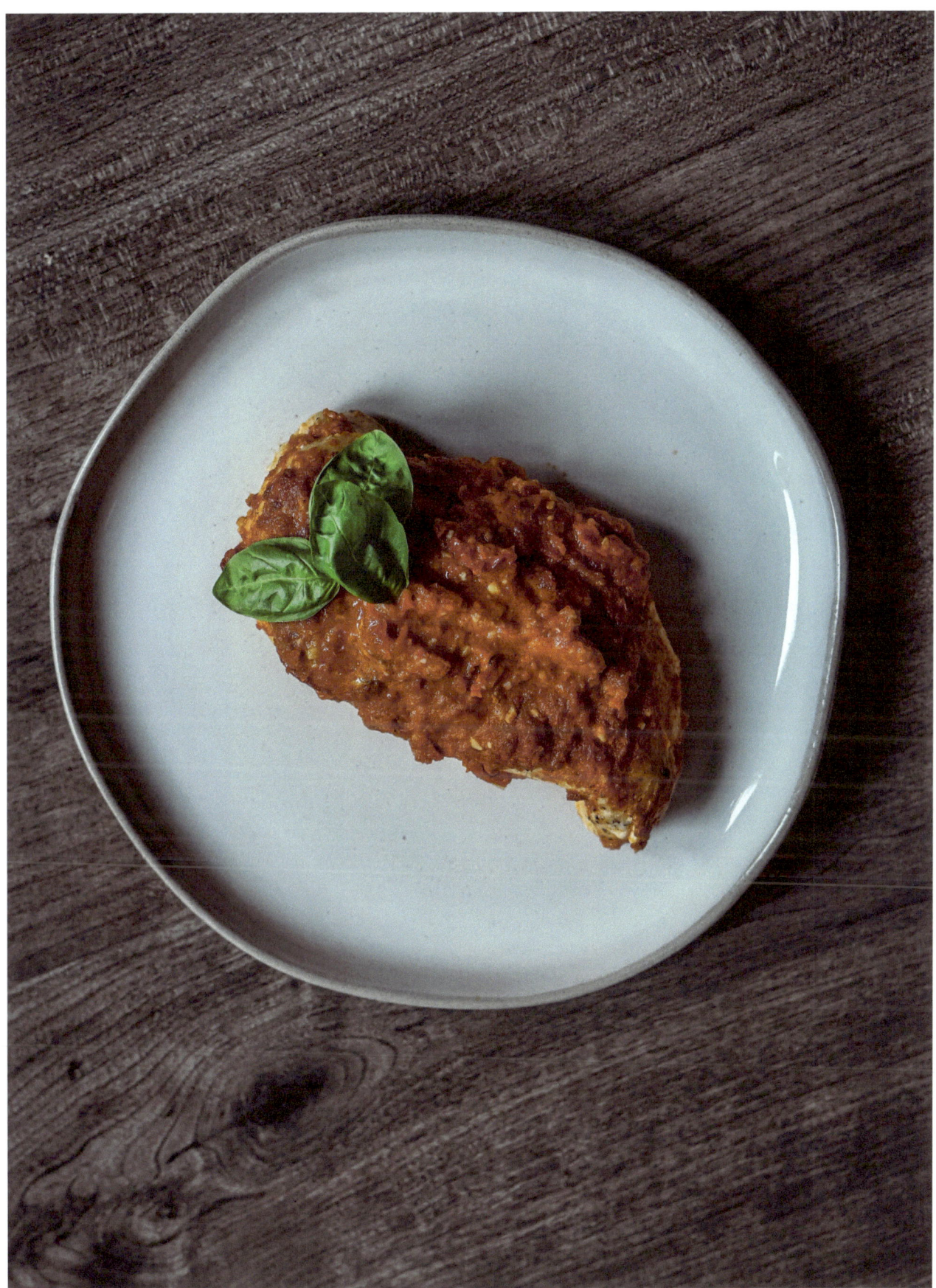

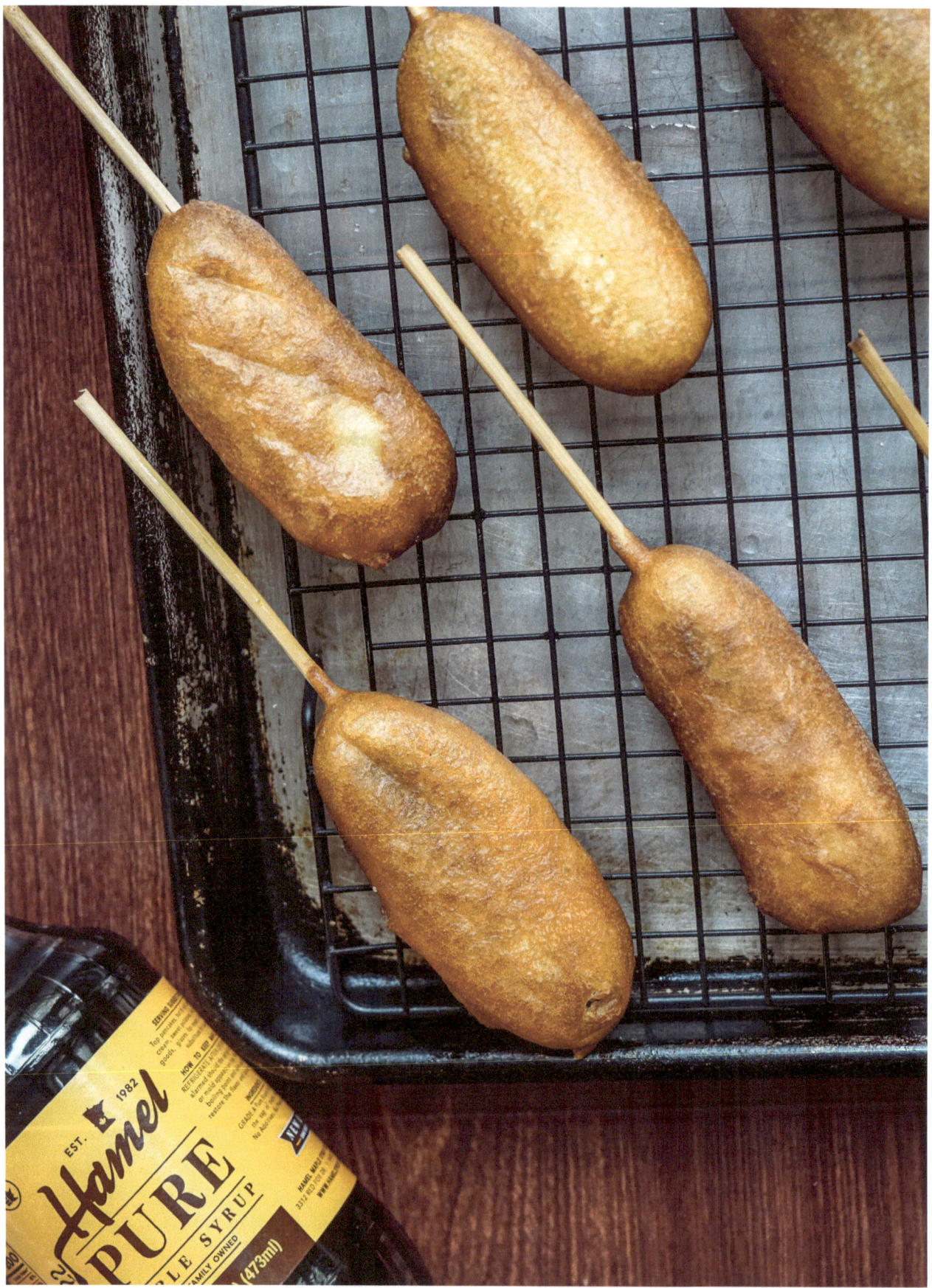

FEELING MYSELF

BREAKFAST BFFS

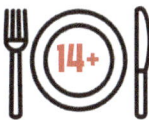

A BUNCH
(DEPENDS ON HOW MANY SAUSAGES YOU HAVE)
14+

PAIRS WELL WITH:
- BACHELORETTE BRUNCHES
- VATS OF MAPLE SYRUP
- SWEET + SALTY CRAVINGS

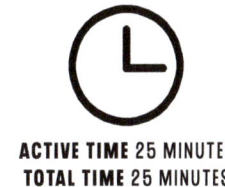

ACTIVE TIME 25 MINUTES
TOTAL TIME 25 MINUTES

SPECIAL EQUIPMENT

7 wood skewers, cut in half
Meat or candy thermometer
Kitchen tongs
Paper towels
Clothing you don't care about (for frying)

INGREDIENTS

1 Tablespoon canola oil
1 pound breakfast sausage links
2 cups all purpose flour
1 teaspoon baking soda
1 teaspoon baking powder
1 teaspoon salt
¼ cup sugar
1 ¼ cups milk
2 large eggs
¼ cup melted butter or butter alternative
4 cups canola oil, for frying
Maple syrup, for dipping

SKEWER SWAP

In a pinch, you can use **toothpicks** and smaller sausage pieces to make mini breakfast buddies.

INSTRUCTIONS

COOK THE SAUSAGE

Heat a pan on the stove over medium heat, then add one tablespoon canola oil.

As the oil heats up, place the sausage links in the pan, leaving a midwestern amount of space between them.

Use the kitchen tongs to rotate the links every few minutes until all sides are golden-brown and a little crispy. Once cooked, place the sausages on a plate lined with paper towels and let them cool.

BATTER UP

In a medium bowl whisk together the flour, baking soda, baking powder, salt and sugar. Once complete, make a deep well in the middle of the dry ingredients and add the milk, eggs and melted butter.

Use a spatula or fork to stir the wet and dry ingredients together. The batter should start to thicken at this point, but if it seems a little thin, feel free to add a little flour at a time until it gets thick enough to stick to the sausages.

Pour or scoop the batter into a tall drinking glass until it's about two-thirds full. Set the extra batter aside, but keep it handy for refilling.

ASSEMBLE THE BUDDIES

Insert a skewer into each sausage, being sure to leave a little skewer exposed as a "handle."

Heat the rest of the canola oil in a deep-sided pan, using the thermometer to monitor the temperature of the oil. You're going to want to keep the oil between 330°F and 370°F when frying to avoid burnt or greasy buds, so feel free to adjust the heat setting on the stove accordingly.

Using the exposed wood skewer as a handle, dip each sausage stick into the glass of batter.

Place it into the oil until fully golden brown, (about one minute per side). Using your tongs, grab it and set it onto a cooling rack with a baking sheet under it to catch any excess oil while it cools.

Drizzle with a little maple syrup, then enjoy before you have to share.

FEELING MYSELF

BITCHIN' BIRTHDAY CAKE

MAKES ONE
AWESOME CAKE
(ABOUT 8 SERVINGS)

PAIRS WELL WITH:
- GETTING CHOCOLATE WASTED
- CELEBRATIONS
- PEOPLE WHO THINK
THEY DON'T LIKE CAKE

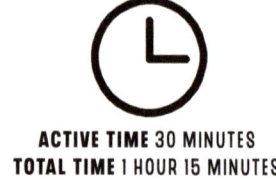

ACTIVE TIME 30 MINUTES
TOTAL TIME 1 HOUR 15 MINUTES

SPECIAL EQUIPMENT

Stand or hand mixer
Cake pan (1 for single tier, 2 for two-tier)
Spatula or butter knife

INGREDIENTS

CAKE
2 cups flour
1 ¾ cups sugar
¾ cup cocoa powder
2 teaspoons baking powder
1 ½ teaspoons baking soda
1 teaspoon salt
½ cup olive oil
2 eggs
1 Tablespoon vanilla
1 cup milk (or coconut milk)
1 cup boiling water - trust us, it'll make sense later

BUTTERCREAM FROSTING
1 cup cocoa powder (unless you want vanilla buttercream)
1 ½ cups (three sticks) room-temperature butter (or butter alternative)
½ cup milk
5 cups powdered sugar
2 teaspoons vanilla

BONUS POINTS
Top with the bourbon bubble sugar for a little extra pizzazz (page 111).

INSTRUCTIONS

Preheat the oven to 350°F and grease the pan(s) you plan to use.

MAKE THE CAKE
In a large bowl combine the flour, sugar, cocoa, baking powder, baking soda and salt.

Add the oil, eggs, vanilla and milk and mix at a medium speed for one to two minutes until well incorporated.

Turn the mixer speed to low, then slowly pour the boiling water into the bowl. Gradually increase the speed until the water is well-mixed into the batter. The batter will be pretty runny at this point, which is exactly what we want!

Pour the batter evenly into the pan(s) and bake for 30-35 minutes, until a knife can be inserted into the center and come out clean.

FROST IT
Wash the large bowl you used earlier, then dump in the cocoa powder. Add the butter to the bowl and mix until nice and creamy.

Add half the milk and half the powdered sugar to the bowl and mix until smooth.

Pour in the vanilla, the other half of the milk, and the powdered sugar, then continue mixing.

Time to check in. Too dry? Add a bit more milk. Too wet? Add a bit more powdered sugar.

We recommend starting on a low speed, then gradually increasing until you get a fluffy frosting. As you increase speed, more air will get incorporated into the frosting and the color will brighten.

Once out of the oven, let the cake cool in the pan for about five minutes, then transfer onto a cooling rack. If we don't let it cool completely before frosting, the cake will melt all the butter, resulting in a puddle of delicious chaos.

STACK IT
If you're making a multi-layer cake you'll want to trim the bottom cake (to make it flat), add a layer of frosting, then place the other cake on top.

Frost the whole thing, slice, and sink into chocolatey deliciousness.

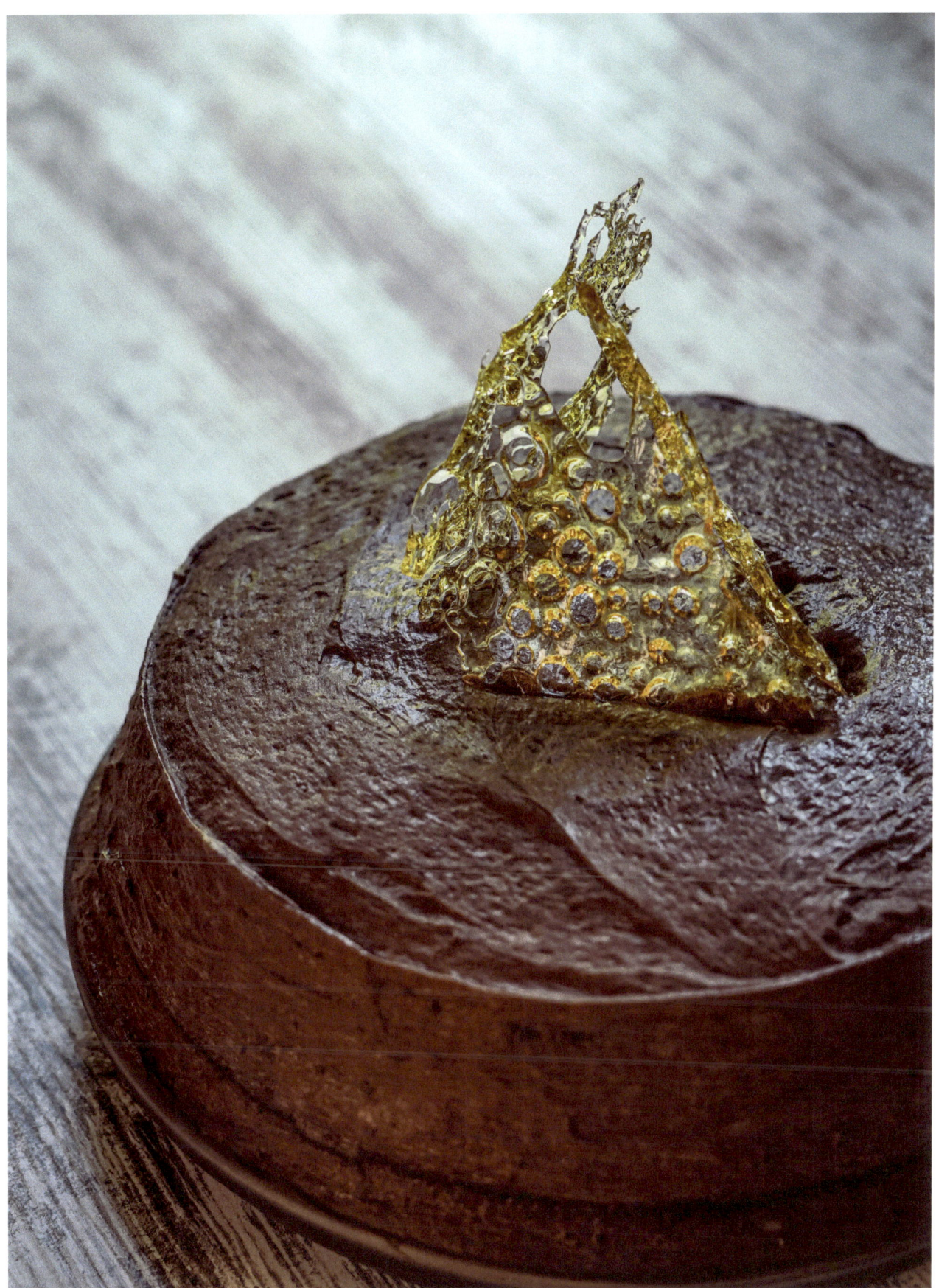

FEELING MYSELF
BOURBON BUBBLE SUGAR

MAKES 1 SWEET SHEET

PAIRS WELL WITH:
- FANCY PANTS
- DESSERTS IN NEED OF FLAIR
- BOURBON BUFFS

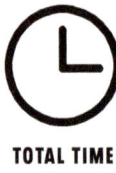

TOTAL TIME
15 MINUTES

HERE'S THE DEAL
The sugar will pick up color, flavor, and fun bubbles from the alcohol!

We chose bourbon, but feel free to swap in any liquor you like for a fantastic addition to any dessert.

SPECIAL EQUIPMENT
- Candy thermometer
- Parchment paper

INGREDIENTS
- ¾ cup sugar
- 1 ½ Tablespoons corn syrup
- ½ cup water
- 2 Tablespoons bourbon

INSTRUCTIONS
- Cut a piece of parchment paper the same size as your baking sheet. Crumple it into a ball, half-heartedly flatten it out onto the sheet, and set aside.
- In a small saucepan, combine the sugar, corn syrup and water over medium-high heat.
- Stir until the sugar dissolves, then place the candy thermometer into the saucepan and cook, stirring regularly until it reaches 315°F.
- While the sugar mixture heats, pour the bourbon onto the baking sheet and spread it around until the parchment is fully coated.
- When the contents of the saucepan hit 315°F, remove the pan from the heat and pour the liquid evenly over the bourbon on the parchment, holding the pan at an angle so the sugar flows down the parchment.
- Let the candy cool until it hardens, then peel away the parchment, crack the sugar apart, and add it to your dessert. Or your stomach.

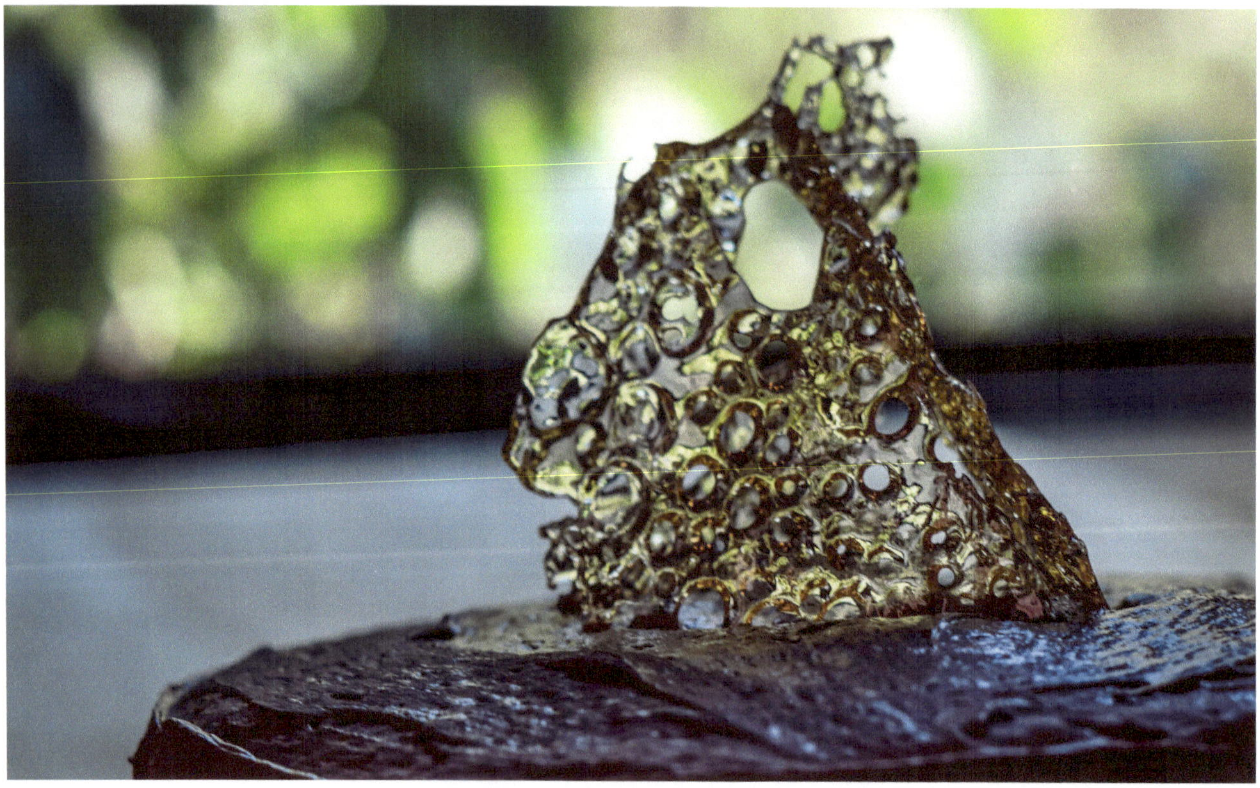

GF DF V

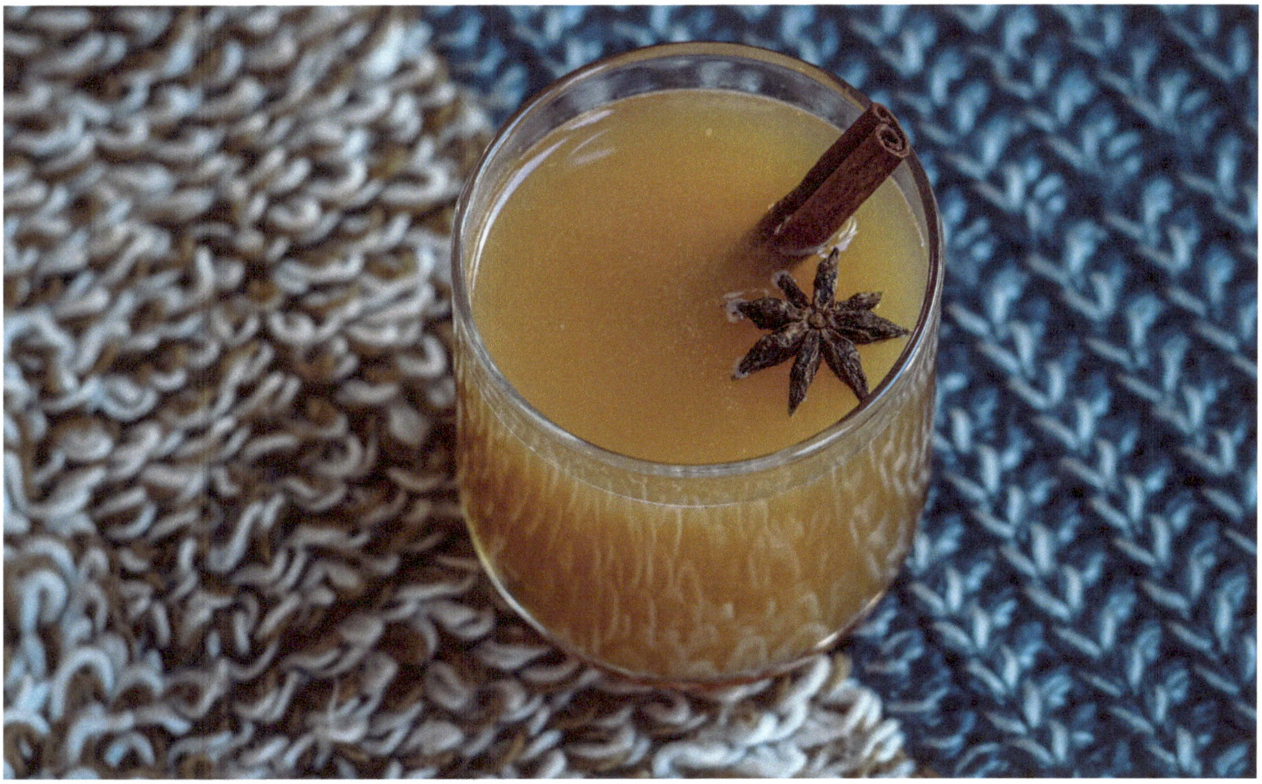

MULLED CIDER

MAKES 1 GALLON (16 GLASSES)

PAIRS WELL WITH:
- ROSY CHEEKS
- CROONER PLAYLISTS
- HEAT UP, WINDOWS DOWN

ACTIVE TIME 5 MINUTES
TOTAL TIME 4 HOURS

SPECIAL EQUIPMENT
Cheesecloth, reusable tea bag, or coffee filter

INGREDIENTS
- 1 gallon apple cider
- 2 cinnamon sticks
- 1 teaspoon whole cloves
- 4 star anise pods
- ½ teaspoon allspice berries
- 1 inch knob of ginger, skin removed and sliced thin
- 1 ½ cups bourbon, brandy or dark rum (if you're feeling it)
- Orange slices, for garnish

INSTRUCTIONS
- Toss all of the spices (cinnamon, cloves, star anise, and allspice) into a pan.
- Toast the spices over medium heat until your kitchen smells amazing (about two minutes), stirring them frequently to avoid burning.
- Remove the spices from heat and put them in a reusable tea bag, cheesecloth or coffee filter.
- Pour the cider into a crockpot or stock pot, then toss in the bag of spices and cover.
- Turn to high heat (if using a crock pot) or low heat (for a stock pot), then let the cider and spice flavors meld together for about four hours.
- Pull out the spices, add the liquor 10-15 minutes before serving, and enjoy!

WORD TO THE WISE
If you add the booze too early, the alcohol will evaporate, so we recommend keeping an eye on timing if you want a buzz!

FEELING MYSELF

BEES KNEES

MAKES 1 DRINK

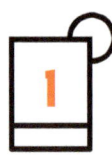

PAIRS WELL WITH:
- SHOWING OFF YOUR ANKLES, YOU MINX
- DECADENT GLASSES
- BEE FREAKS

TOTAL TIME
5 MINUTES

SPECIAL EQUIPMENT
Cocktail shaker

INGREDIENTS
- ½ ounce homemade honey syrup (sounds hard, but isn't)
- 2 ounces gin
- ¾ ounce fresh-squeezed lemon juice
- Lemon twist garnish (optional)
- Ice

INSTRUCTIONS

MAKE THE SYRUP FIRST, HONEY.
Mix equal parts honey and water in a small saucepan over medium heat. You want the mixture to get warm, but don't let it boil! Stir until the honey dissolves, then set it aside to cool.

THE DRINK
- Measure a half-ounce of honey syrup into a shaker over ice.
- Top with gin and lemon juice, then shake until cold (about 30 seconds).
- Pour into a chilled glass, garnish however you like, and serve.

LEMON TWIST 101
Cut one circular lemon slice, then use a knife to cut through the peel on one side of the circle. Trim away all the fruit from the inside of the slice, leaving a (circular) strip of lemon rind. Twist this rind into a little pig tail (or twist) and you're all set! This technique can be used with any variety of citrus.

Now go show off to your friends!

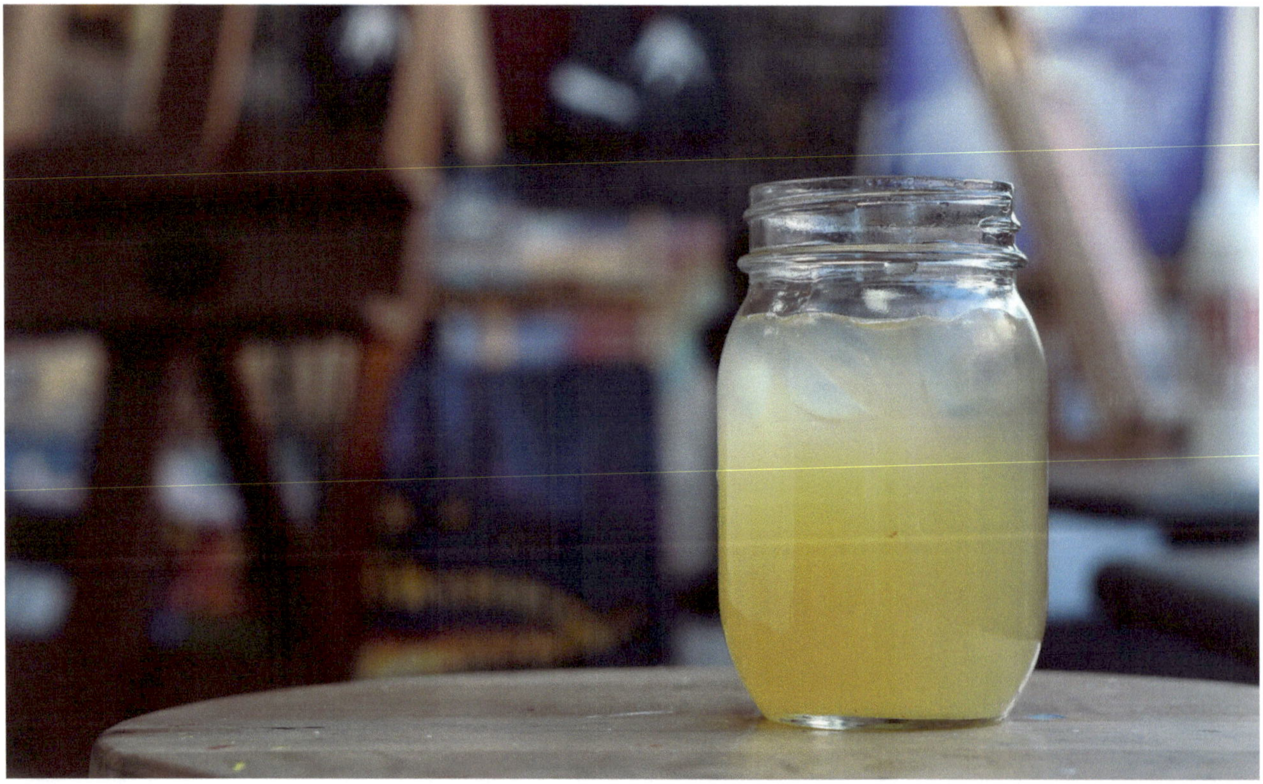

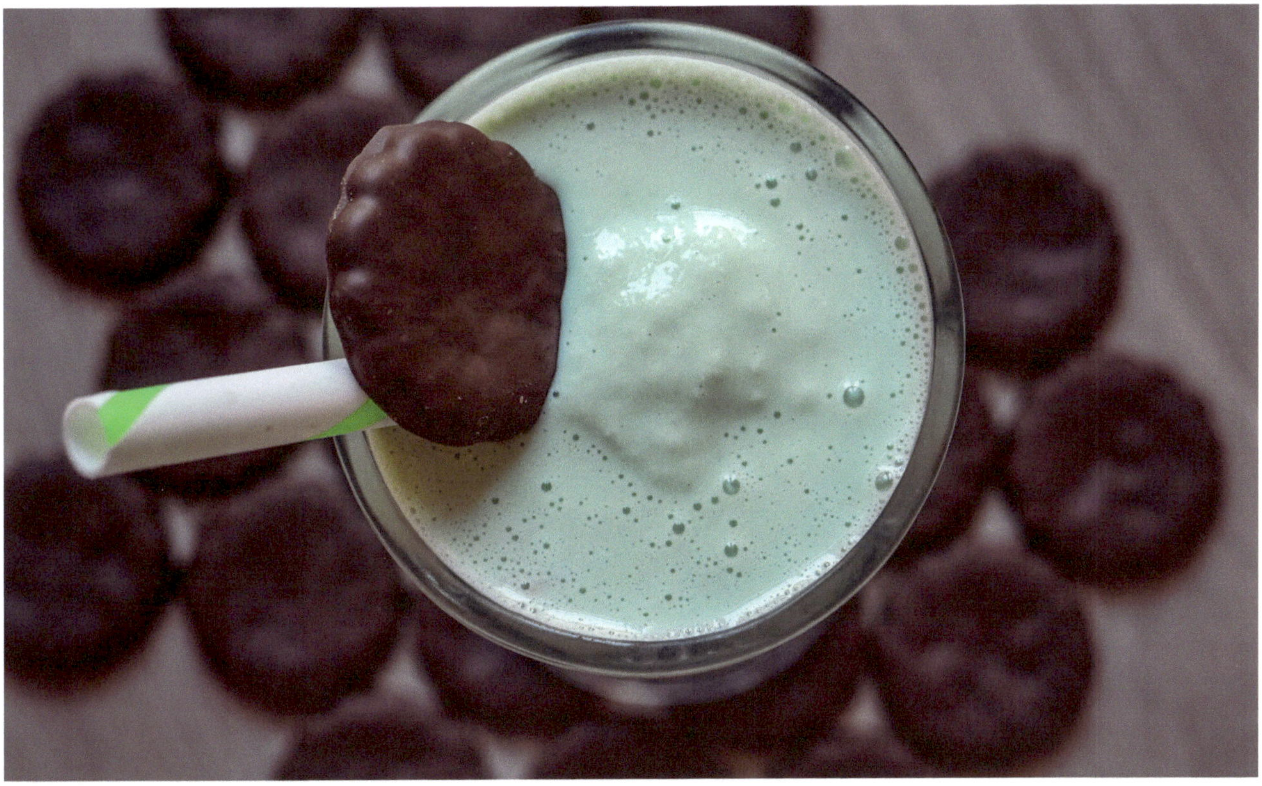

GOOD DAY GRASSHOPPER

MAKES 1 INDULGENT DESSERT OR 2 DRINKS

PAIRS WELL WITH:
- TREATING YOURSELF FOR NO REASON AT ALL
- SERIOUS COOKIE CRAVINGS
- LOST TOOTHBRUSHES

TOTAL TIME
5 MINUTES

SPECIAL EQUIPMENT
Blender

INGREDIENTS
- 1 pint mint chocolate chip ice cream (you can substitute vanilla in a pinch)
- ½ cup milk
- 1 ½ ounces Creme de Cacao
- 1 ½ ounces Creme de Menthe

SERVE WITH
- Chocolate syrup
- Mint cookies
- Whipped cream
- Maraschino cherry

INSTRUCTIONS
- Toss the ice cream, milk, and booze into a blender.
- Pulse until smooth (about 15-30 seconds).
- Pour into a tall glass and top with unapologetic sweetness - cookies, chocolate syrup, whipped cream, cherries...you name it.

FEELING

PANICKED

FEELING PANICKED

GOAT CHEESE + APRICOT CROSTINI

MAKES AT LEAST 4 SERVINGS

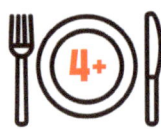

PAIRS WELL WITH:
- IMPROMPTU PARTIES
- RAPID GROCERY RUNS
- PICNICS

ACTIVE TIME
5 MINUTES
TOTAL TIME
10 MINUTES

INGREDIENTS
- 1 french baguette
- 1 container spreadable goat cheese
- 1 jar apricot preserves
- ½ cup crushed pistachios
- Fresh mint for garnish

INSTRUCTIONS
- Start by preheating your oven to 400°F.
- Cut the bread into ¼-½ inch slices.
- Lay the slices flat on a baking sheet.
- Put them in the oven for five minutes, just long enough to toast the tops.
- Remove from the oven and spread a smear of goat cheese onto the bread, followed by the apricot preserves and a sprinkle of pistachios.
- Top with a mint leaf or two and place on a nice serving dish.

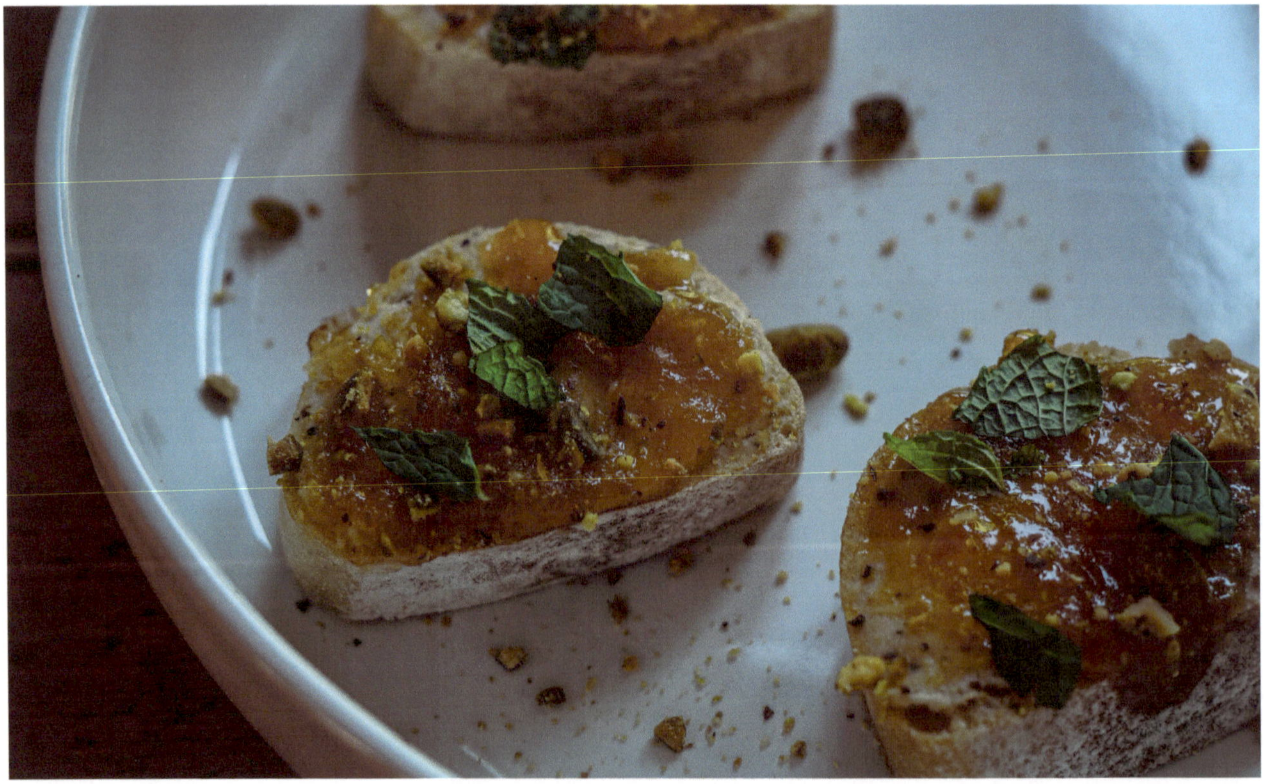

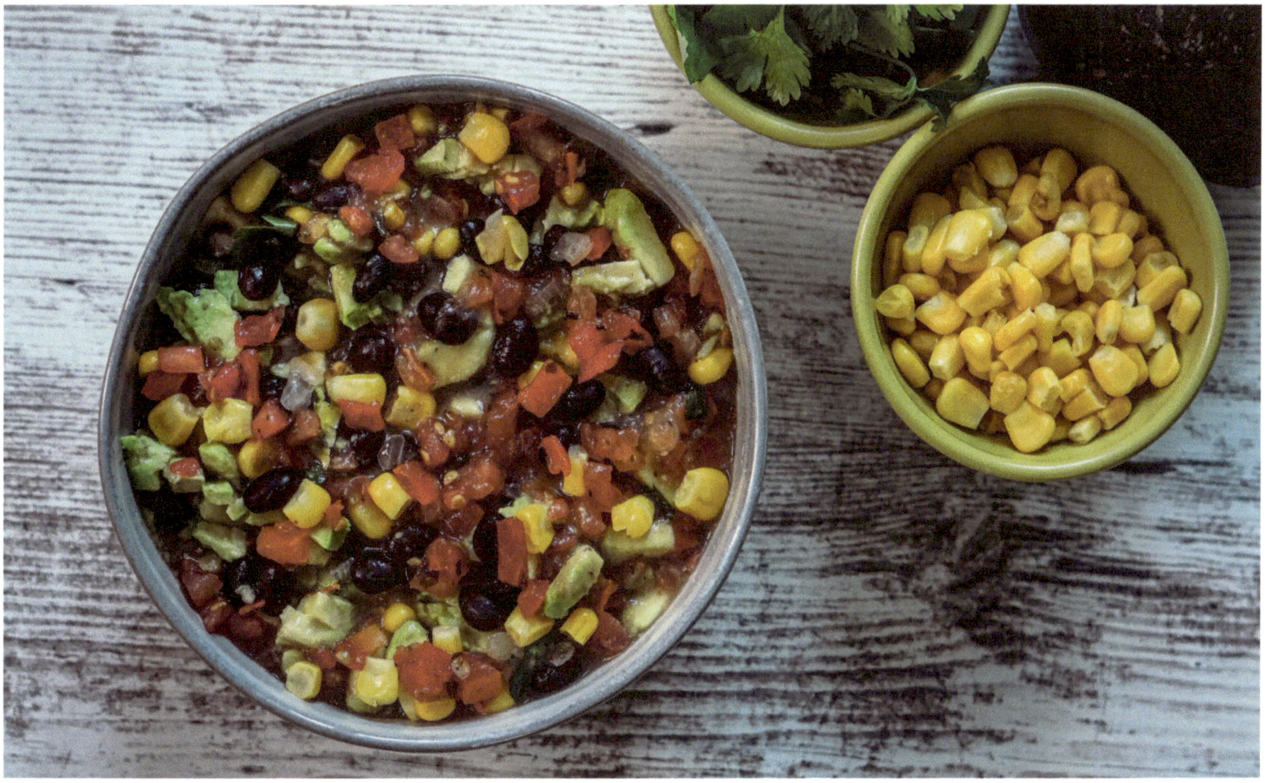

WARP-SPEED SALSA DIP

MAKES 4 CUPS

PAIRS WELL WITH:
- UNINVITED GUESTS
- PINEAPPLE MARGARITAS
- BACKYARD GARDENS

TOTAL TIME
5 MINUTES

INGREDIENTS
- 16 ounces premade pico de gallo or other salsa from your grocery store
- ½ cup canned corn
- ½ cup canned black beans
- ¼ cup cilantro, chopped
- 2 Tablespoons lime juice
- 1 ripe avocado

HERE'S THE DEAL

Think of the ingredient measurements as guidelines rather than rules.

Corn adds sweetness, beans add bulk, cilantro adds a soapy taste (jk but know your audience) and lime juice adds zest.

INSTRUCTIONS
- Toss the fresh salsa in a large bowl.
- Stir in the corn, black beans, cilantro, and lime juice.
- Cut the avocado in half, slice the guts into small chunks, and add them to the salsa.
- Mix lightly (the more you mix, the creamier the salsa will get).
- Serve with tortilla chips.

FEELING PANICKED

EASY AFRICAN PEANUT SOUP

MAKES 4 BOWLS OF SOUP

PAIRS WELL WITH:
- PEOPLE YOU DON'T KNOW (THIS ONE'S A CROWD PLEASER)
- PB FREAKS
- CRUSTY BREAD

ACTIVE TIME 10 MINUTES
TOTAL TIME 40 MINUTES

SPECIAL EQUIPMENT

One large pot

INGREDIENTS

4 cups vegetable broth
2 cups water
1 large red onion, chopped
2 inch chunk (or 2 knobs) ginger, minced
5 cloves garlic, minced
1 teaspoon salt
¾ cup peanut butter
½ cup tomato paste
1 bunch kale, chopped or torn, stems removed
1 teaspoon sriracha or similar hot sauce (adjust for your heat preference)

SERVE WITH

Brown rice
Chopped peanuts (for garnish)

INSTRUCTIONS

Pour the vegetable broth and water into a stock pot, then bring to a boil over high heat.

Add the onion, ginger, garlic and salt, then reduce to a simmer (medium-low) for about 20 minutes.

While the pot simmers, measure the peanut butter and tomato paste into a medium-sized bowl.

Stir 1 ½ cups of the stock into the peanut-butter-tomato combo until smooth.

Once the remaining stock has simmered for 20 minutes, toss the peanut butter mix into the pot along with the kale and hot sauce and stir.

Simmer for another 15 minutes.

Taste, adjust the heat and salt to suit your taste buds, and you're ready to serve.

Serve the soup alone or spoon it over rice and garnish with chopped peanuts. Yum!

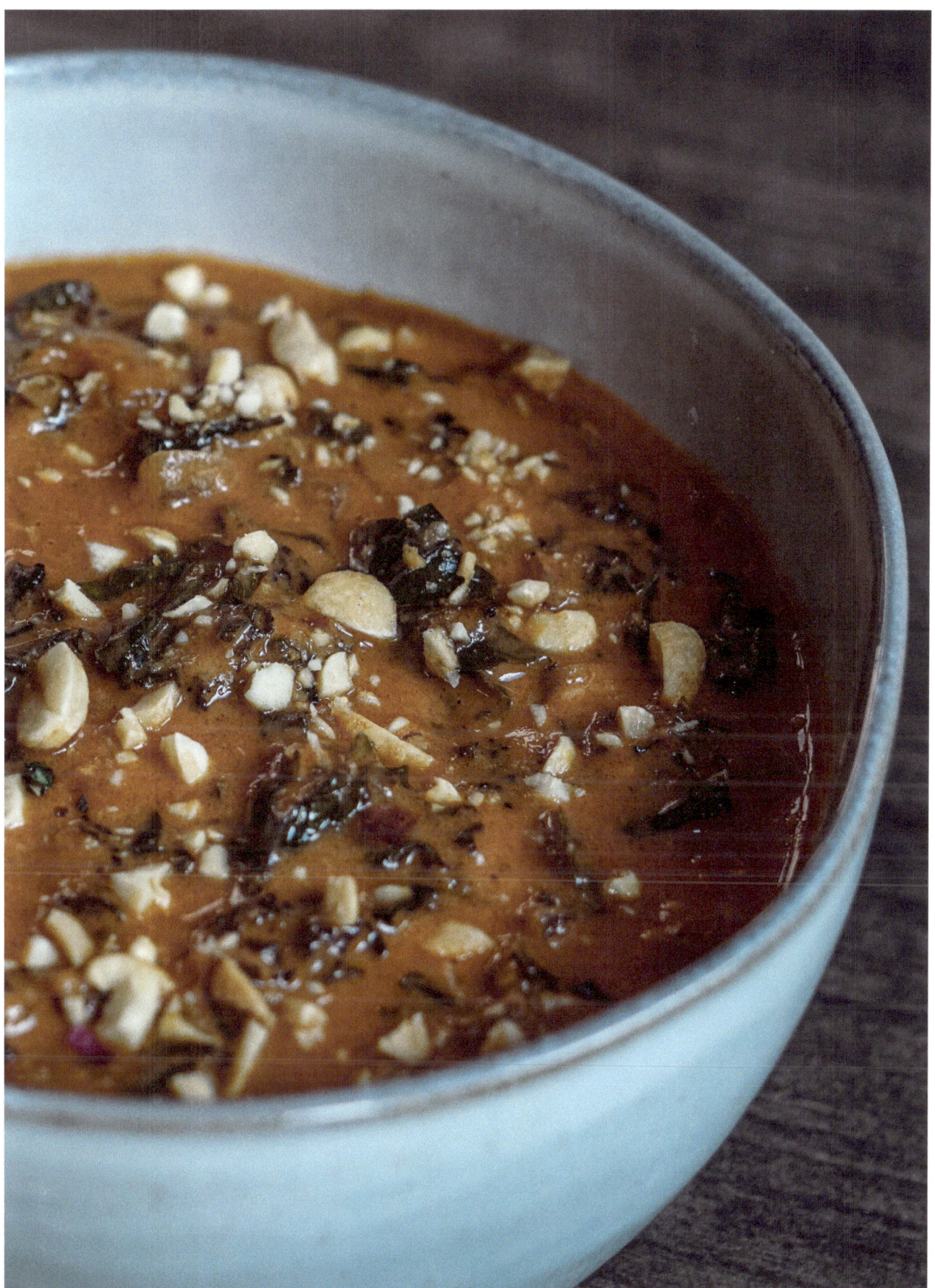

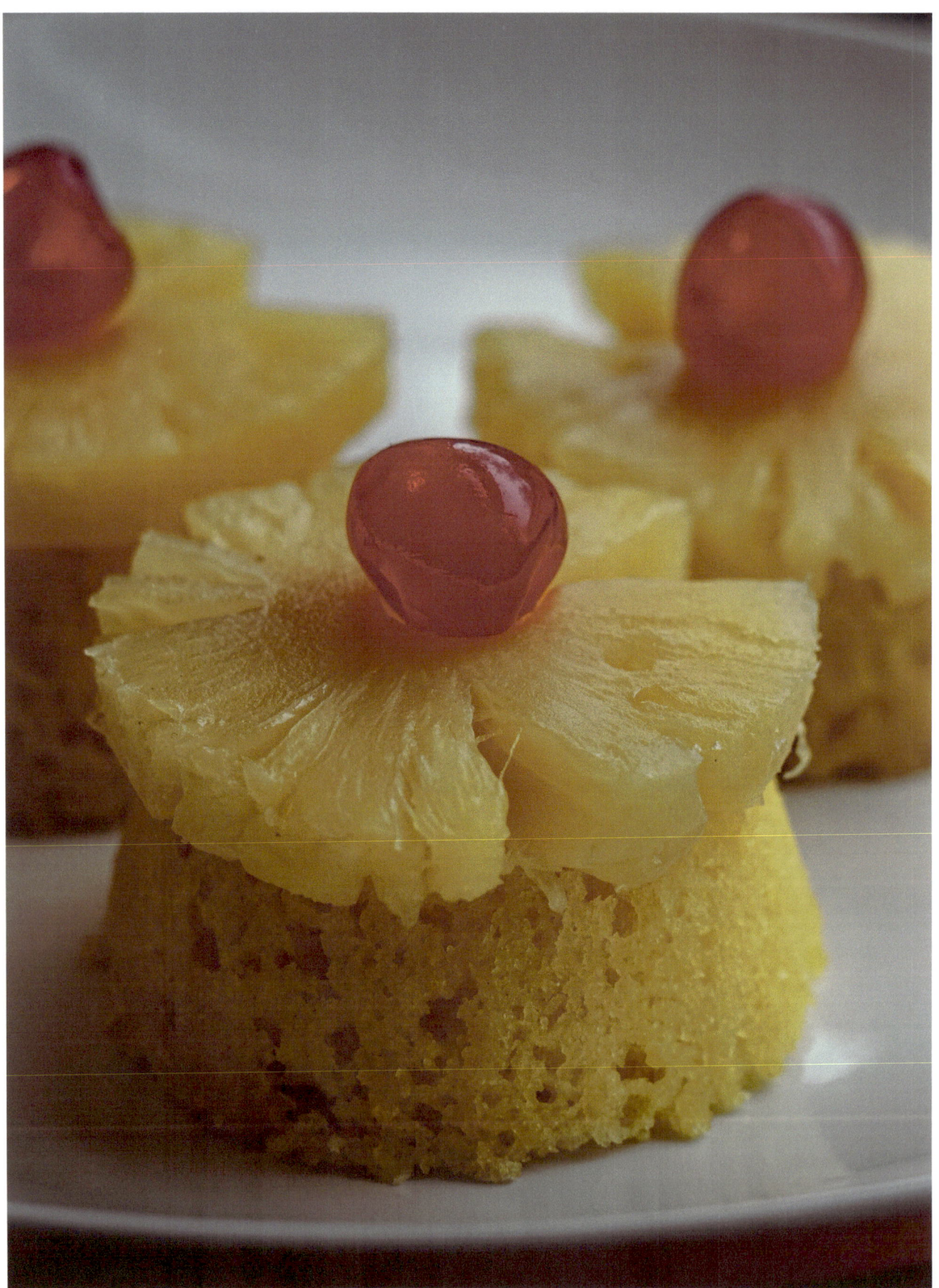

FEELING PANICKED

QUICK LITTLE PINEAPPLE CAKES

MAKES 24 MINI CAKES

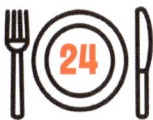

PAIRS WELL WITH:
- FAMILY REUNIONS
- THAT PINEAPPLE IN THE BACK OF YOUR PANTRY
- TINY HELPING HANDS

ACTIVE TIME 5 MINUTES
TOTAL TIME ABOUT 20 MINUTES
(ASK THE BOX)

SPECIAL EQUIPMENT

Muffin tin
Cooling rack

INGREDIENTS

1 box yellow cake mix
Egg, oil and water (per box instructions)
1 jar maraschino cherries
2 cans sliced pineapple, in its own juice

HERE'S THE DEAL

Though this isn't the original way to make pineapple upside down cake, it looks better than the dried-out pineapple version and doesn't require as much hand-eye coordination.

INSTRUCTIONS

Preheat the oven to the required temperature on the cake mix box.

Separate the pineapple fruit from the juice and set both aside.

Prepare the cake batter according to box instructions with one adjustment: use pineapple juice instead of water!

Use as much pineapple juice as you can get away with (per the liquid recommendation on the box of cake mix), then supplement with water as needed. This will ensure your cake has a light, delicious pineapple flavor from the start.

Grease a muffin tin.

Pour the batter evenly into the pan, filling each cup about ¾ full, then bake per box directions (usually about 15 minutes).

Once the cakes are baked, remove from them oven and let them rest for a minute or two.

Use a butter knife to separate the sides of each muffin from the pan, then use the same knife to cut the tops of the cakes off so they sit even to the surface of the tin.

Place a cutting board over the top of the muffin tin. Hold on tight to the edges and quickly flip the tin over to release the cakes onto the board.

Transfer the cakes to the cooling rack.

Place a slice of pineapple on each cake, put a cherry on top, and serve!

FEELING PANICKED

PAN-FRIED GNOCCHI

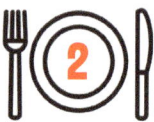

MAKES 2 BOWLS

PAIRS WELL WITH:
- VEGETARIAN GUESTS
- WHITE WINE
- MINIMIZING THE DISHES

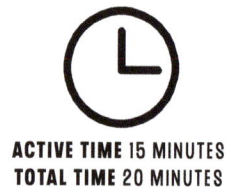

ACTIVE TIME 15 MINUTES
TOTAL TIME 20 MINUTES

SPECIAL EQUIPMENT

Small saucepan
Fry pan

INGREDIENTS

4 cloves garlic, minced
4 sprigs fresh rosemary, chopped
12 ounces brussel sprouts, cut in half
¼ cup pine nuts or walnuts
4 Tablespoons vegetable oil
1 package gnocchi (18 ounces)
¼ cup freshly grated parmesan
Salt to taste

INSTRUCTIONS

Prep the garlic, rosemary, and brussel sprouts.

THE BRUSSELS

Warm a pan over medium heat and toss in the pine nuts or walnuts, being sure to stir them constantly to avoid any burns. Toast the nuts until golden and aromatic, (about two minutes), then remove them from the pan and set aside.

Add two tablespoons of oil to the pan you just used, add the garlic and rosemary and sauté over medium until lightly golden brown. Once golden, remove from the pan and set aside for a few minutes. We will get back to it, we promise.

Add the brussel sprout halves to the pan, flat-side down.

Cook until the brussel sprouts start to brown (about three to five minutes), then stir and cook for an additional three minutes until tender and crispy. Place in a bowl and set aside.

THE GNOCCHI

In the same pan you've been working with this whole time, heat two tablespoons oil over medium-high and add the gnocchi, breaking up any clusters with a spatula. Cover the pan and cook until golden on one side (about two to four minutes). Shake the pan to show a new side of the gnocchi and continue to cook another two minutes until golden brown.

Add all the brussel sprouts, rosemary and garlic into the gnocchi pan over medium-low heat. Stir until everything is coated and warm. Season to taste with salt and pepper and plate the food. Top with freshly grated parmesan, toasted pine nuts and a drizzle of olive oil.

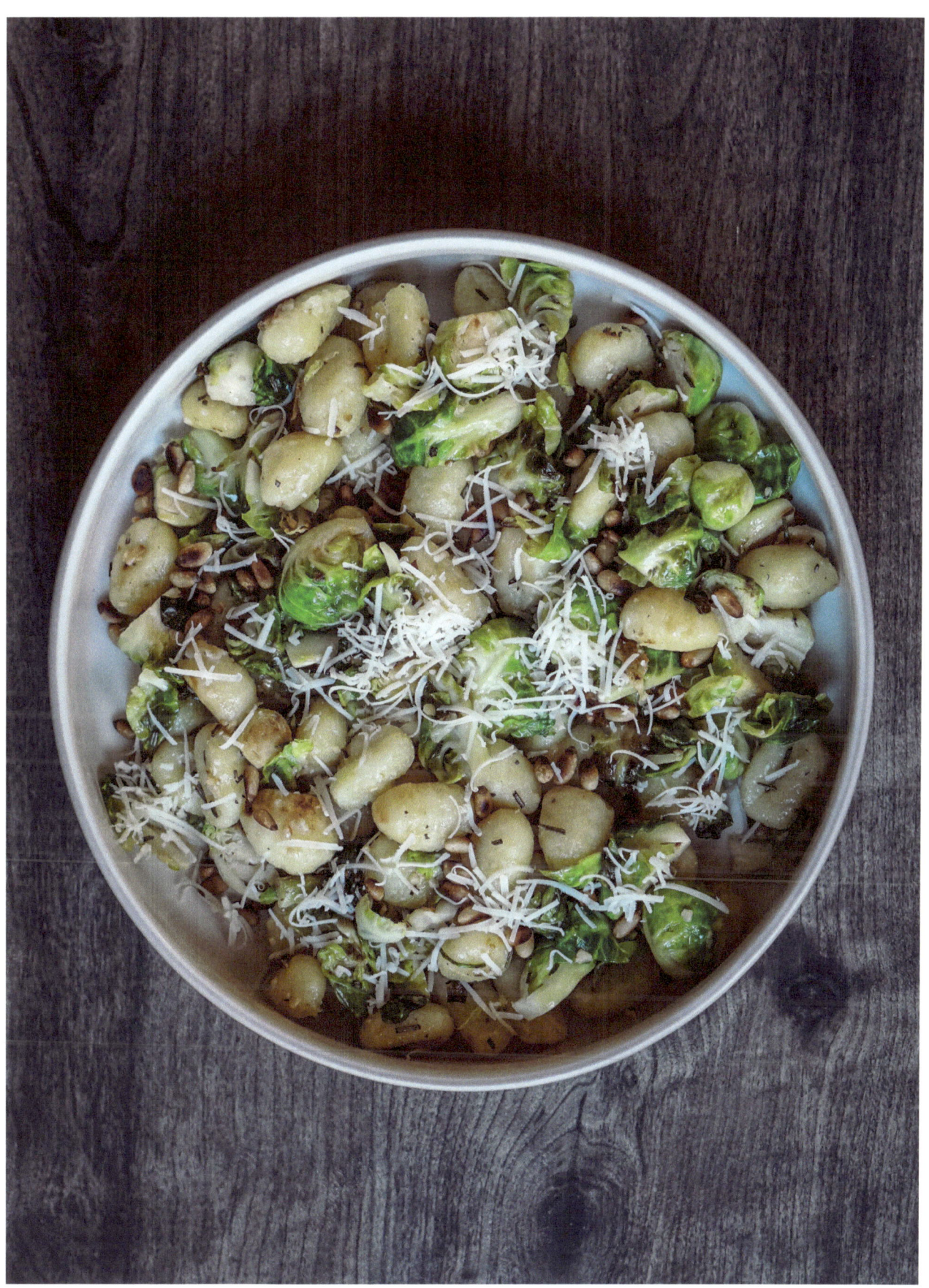

FEELING PANICKED
SPEEDY GRILLED SHRIMP

MAKES 1 POUND (ABOUT 4 SERVINGS)

PAIRS WELL WITH:
- NO TIME FOR TABLE SETTING
- HEAVY BREAKFASTS
- SELF-PROCLAIMED GRILL MASTERS

ACTIVE TIME
15 MINUTES
TOTAL TIME
45 MINUTES

SPECIAL EQUIPMENT
Grill
Large resealable bag

INGREDIENTS
- 1 pound large raw shrimp
- ½ cup orange juice
- ¼ cup olive oil
- ¼ cup brown sugar
- 2 teaspoon Old Bay seasoning
- 1 teaspoon dried minced onion
- ½ teaspoon garlic powder
- ½ teaspoon sage
- ¼ teaspoon black pepper

INSTRUCTIONS
- Defrost, peel & rinse shrimp.
- Combine all ingredients in a large resealable bag & marinate shrimp for 30 minutes.
- Grill on high heat until opaque (about two or three minutes per side).
- Serve with grilled veggies, salad, or whatever else you have on hand.

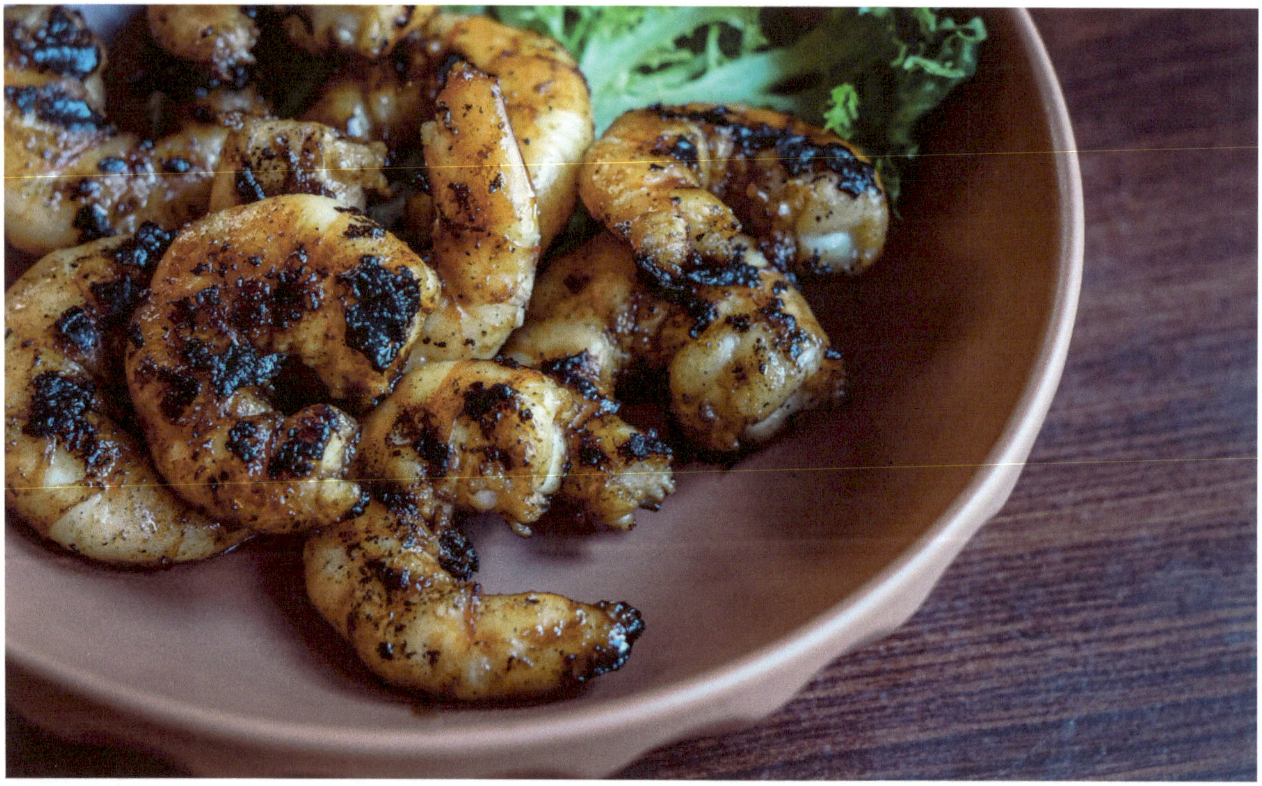

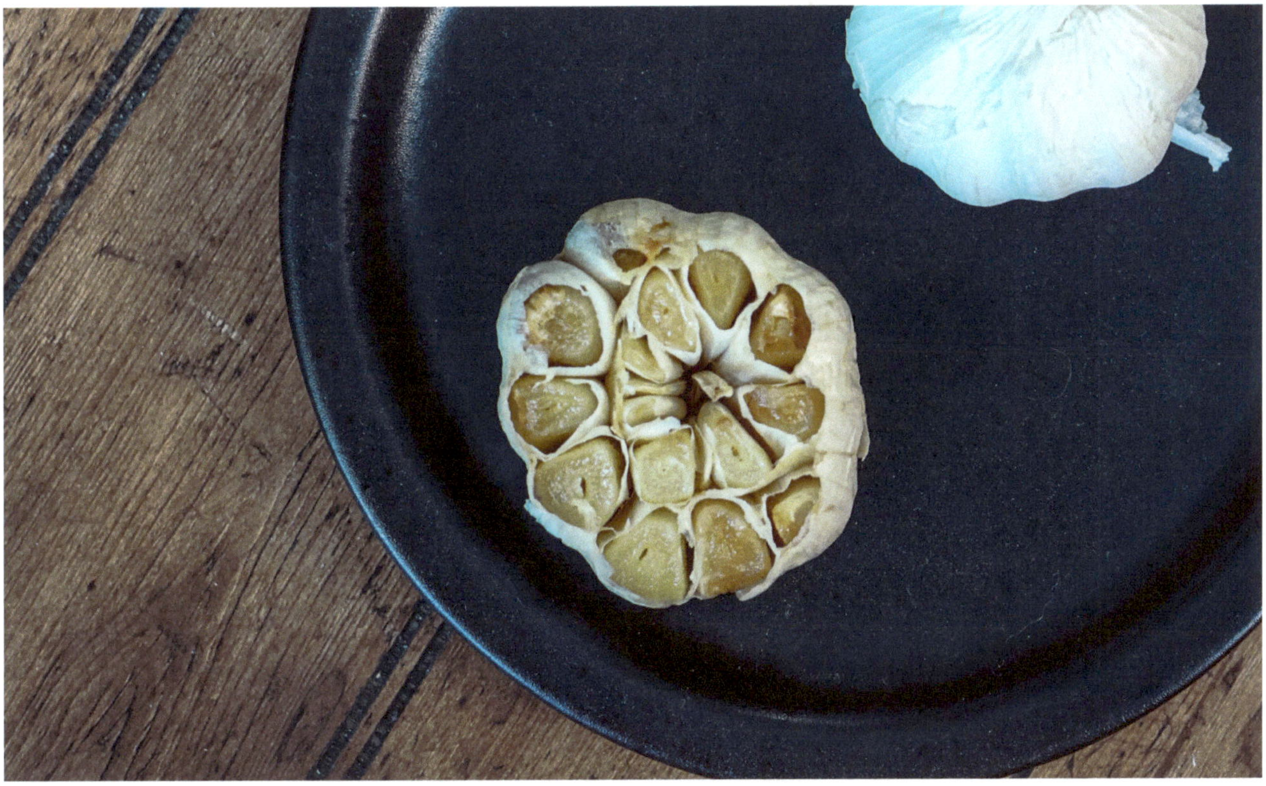

AROMATIC ROASTED GARLIC

MAKES AS MUCH GARLIC AS YOU WANT

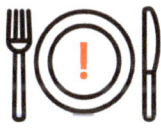

PAIRS WELL WITH:
- NEGLECTED CHORES
- BREAD AND OLIVE OIL
- SUSPECTED VAMPIRES

ACTIVE TIME
5 MINUTES
TOTAL TIME
45 MINUTES

HERE'S THE DEAL
Make these before a dinner party, in-law visit, or an open house for yummy smells. Serve right away, or stash in the fridge for your next cooking adventure.

SPECIAL EQUIPMENT
Aluminum foil, cut into squares
Baking sheet, any size

INGREDIENTS
- Olive oil
- Whole garlic bulbs

INSTRUCTIONS
- Preheat your oven to 400°F.
- Use a knife to chop the top off of each garlic bulb so you can see the cloves (like cutting the roof off a house), then place each one on a square of foil.
- Drizzle a little olive oil into each bulb, then fully enclose it in the foil like a chocolate kiss.
- Place each foil package on a baking sheet in the oven until the delicious scent takes over your kitchen (about 40 minutes).
- Pull out of the oven and place on a cooling rack.

NOW OR LATER
These can be stored in a baggie in the fridge for a few weeks and used anytime garlic is required.

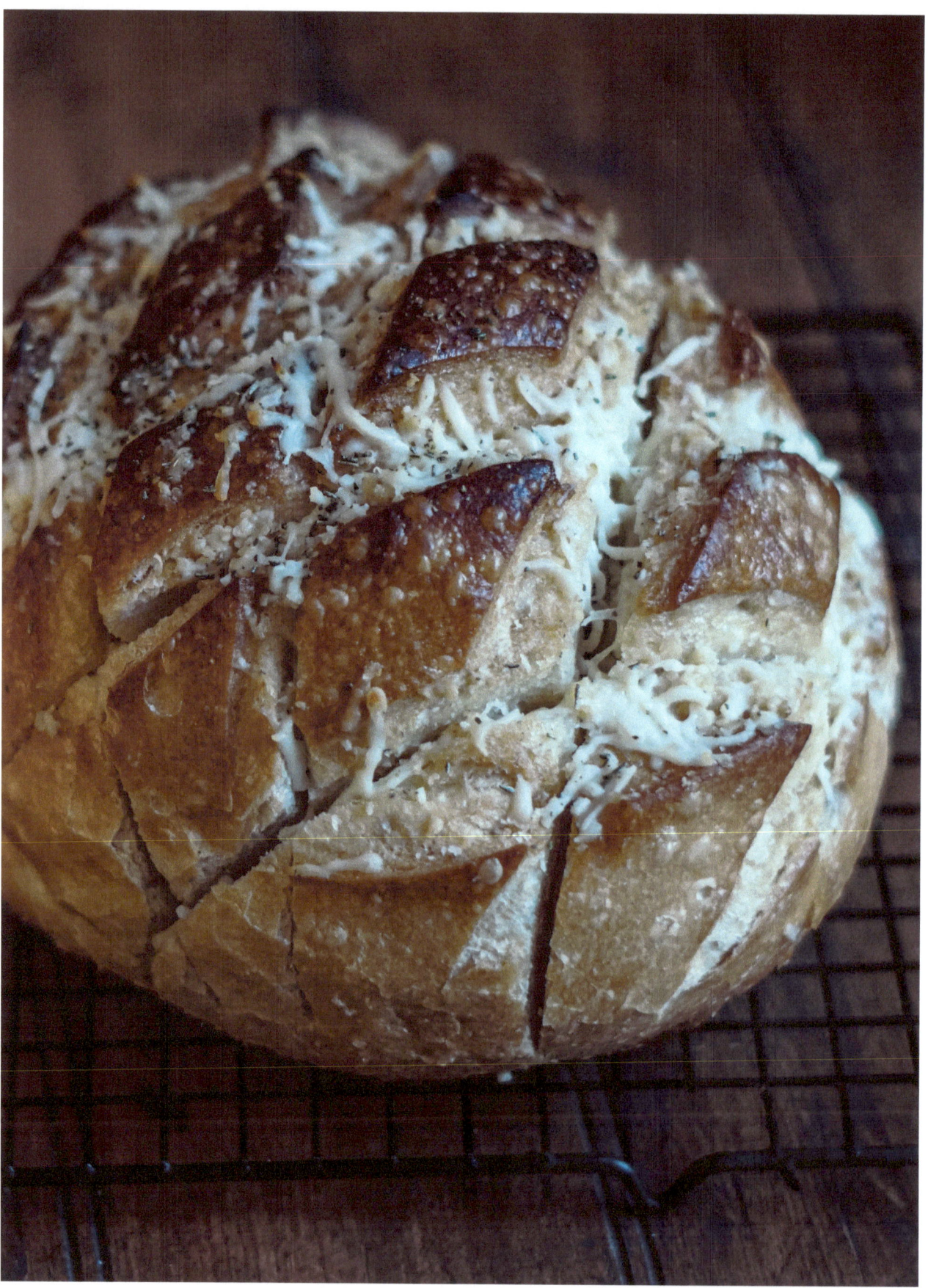

FEELING PANICKED

ROASTED GARLIC PULL-APART BREAD

MAKES 1 LOAF (ABOUT 6-8 SERVINGS)

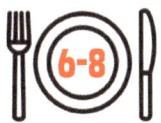

PAIRS WELL WITH:
- STALLING WHILE YOU FIGURE OUT DINNER
- HOMEBODY HAPPY HOUR
- REALLY AWESOME RED SAUCE

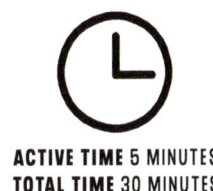

ACTIVE TIME 5 MINUTES
TOTAL TIME 30 MINUTES

INGREDIENTS

1 loaf crusty bread (italian or sourdough are great)
8 Tablespoons butter or butter alternative
3 cloves garlic, minced
1 teaspoon salt
1 Tablespoon rosemary, minced (optional)
1 cup mozzarella cheese (optional)
Marinara sauce (optional)

INSTRUCTIONS

Preheat your oven to 350°F.

Grab the loaf of bread and carefully cut the top into a one-inch square grid, cutting almost all the way to the bottom.

Melt the butter. Once melted, add your garlic, salt and rosemary and stir.

Place the loaf of bread on a baking sheet lined with enough foil to wrap around the bread loaf. Spread each grid line and drizzle in the butter mix about a teaspoon at a time. The deeper it gets, the better the results. Line each grid line with cheese. Finish up by brushing any remaining butter on the top of the loaf and sprinkling with cheese.

Wrap in tinfoil and place in the oven for 15 minutes. Remove from the oven, uncover and return to the oven for five to 10 minutes so the cheese can crisp up and the bread can regain its crustiness.

Remove and serve as is or with a side of marinara sauce.

FEELING PANICKED
SNAPPY AVOCADO + SHRIMP TOAST

MAKES 2 TOASTS

INGREDIENTS
- 1 Tablespoon olive oil
- 4 cloves garlic, minced
- 2 cups medium shrimp, shelled
- ½ cup pre-made guacamole or 1 mashed avocado
- 1 Tablespoon fresh parsley, chopped
- Coarse salt, to taste
- Fresh cracked black pepper, to taste
- 2 slices bread, toasted

INSTRUCTIONS
- Heat a pan over low heat, then add the olive oil.
- Add the garlic and shrimp to the pan, then sprinkle generously with salt.
- Cook until the shrimp is opaque, but not rubbery (no more than five minutes). If you're using pre-cooked shrimp, a quick toss in the warm pan will ensure they are warm but not overcooked.
- Mix the guacamole, shrimp, and parsley together in a bowl, then spoon the mixture generously onto each slice of toast.
- Garnish with parsley, salt, and fresh cracked black pepper and enjoy!

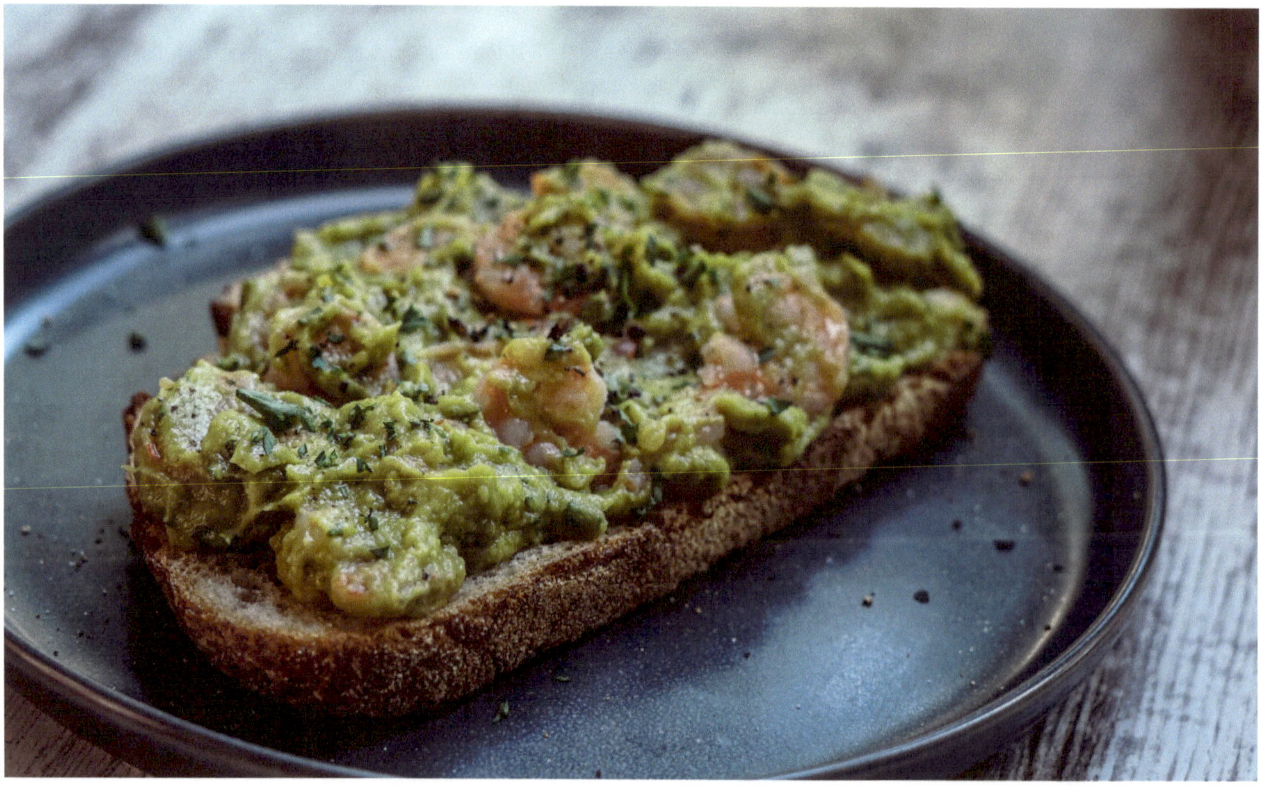

PAIRS WELL WITH:
- QUICK EXITS
- LATE NIGHTS
- STIFF BLOODY MARYS

ACTIVE TIME
5 MINUTES
TOTAL TIME
10 MINUTES

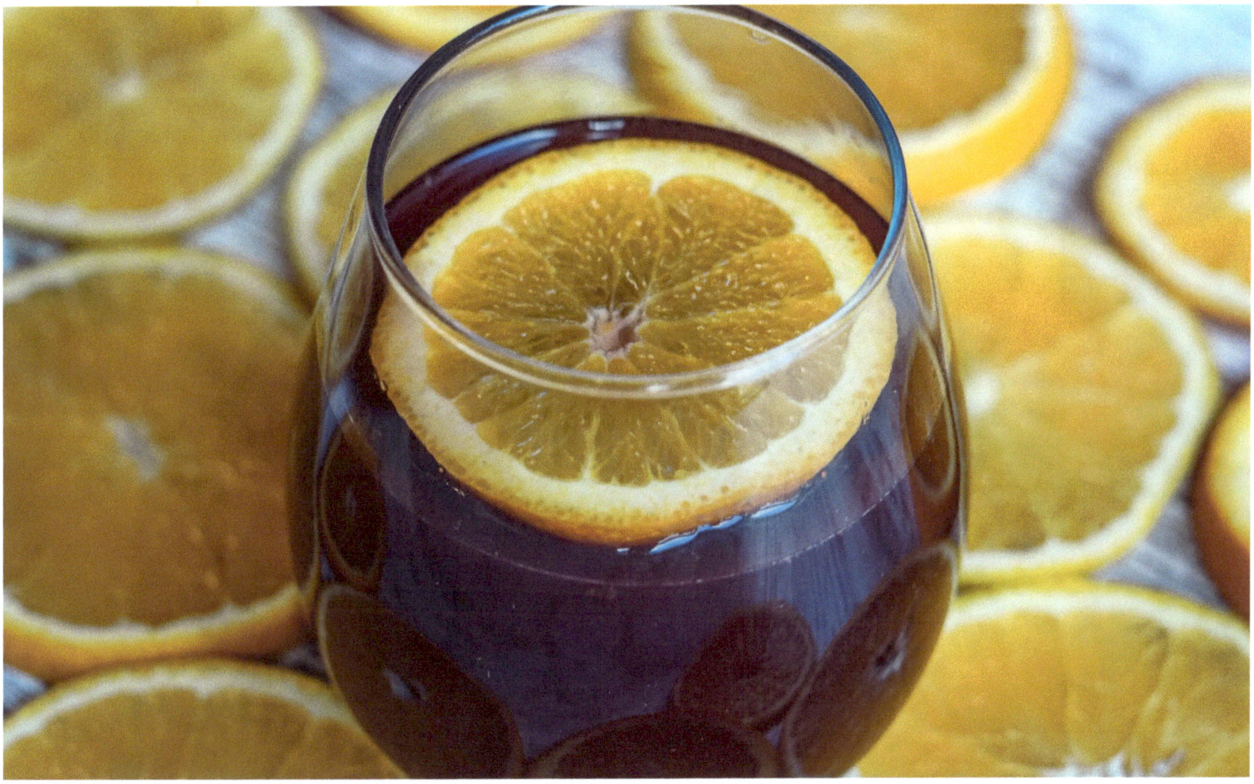

SLAP-TOGETHER SANGRIA

MAKES 6 DRINKS

PAIRS WELL WITH:
- MOTHERS-IN-LAW
- GARDEN PARTIES
- OVERCOMMITTING ON PRODUCE FOR THE WEEK

ACTIVE TIME
5 MINUTES
TOTAL TIME
UP TO 3 HOURS

SPECIAL EQUIPMENT
Large pitcher or punch bowl

INGREDIENTS
- 1 cup orange juice
- ¼ cup orange liqueur (Grand Marnier or Cointreau)
- 1 bottle (750ml) red wine (spanish red, burgundy or pinot noir work great)
- ¼ cup brandy
- 1 ½ cups seasonal fruit, sliced

HERE'S THE DEAL
If you get enough notice to make this ahead of time, we recommend refrigerating it for a few hours. No time? No worries; it will still be delicious slapped together and thrown over ice.

INSTRUCTIONS
- Pop all the ingredients into a large pitcher and stir.
- Pour into glasses and garnish with a slice of fruit.
- Feel free to add ginger ale or seltzer water if you want some bubbles!

FEELING PANICKED

FRENCH 75

MAKES 1 BUBBLY DRINK

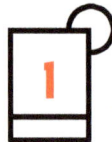

SPECIAL EQUIPMENT
Cocktail shaker

INGREDIENTS
- 1 ½ ounces gin
- ¾ ounce fresh squeezed lemon juice
- ½ ounce simple syrup
- 3 ounces champagne
- Fresh ice
- Lemon twist for garnish (optional)

PAIRS WELL WITH:
- STANDBY CHAMPAGNE
- GOOD NEWS
- PEOPLE WHO LIKE TO GIVE TOASTS

INSTRUCTIONS
- Pour the gin, lemon juice, and simple syrup into a cocktail shaker with a handful of ice.
- Shake until well-combined (about 15 seconds), then strain into a champagne flute.
- Top with champagne, garnish with a lemon twist if you like, and enjoy!

GROUP TIP
You should be able to get about 8 drinks per bottle of champagne.

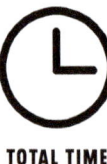

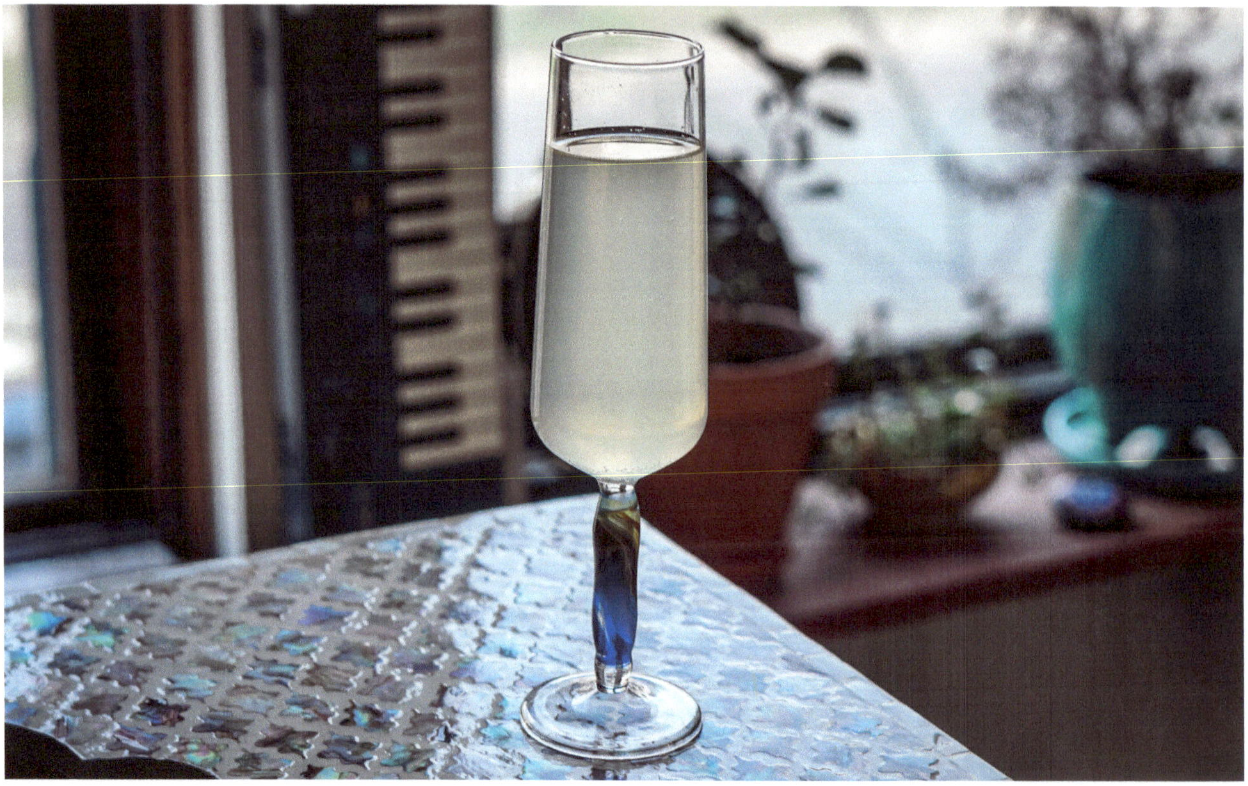

TOTAL TIME
3 MINUTES

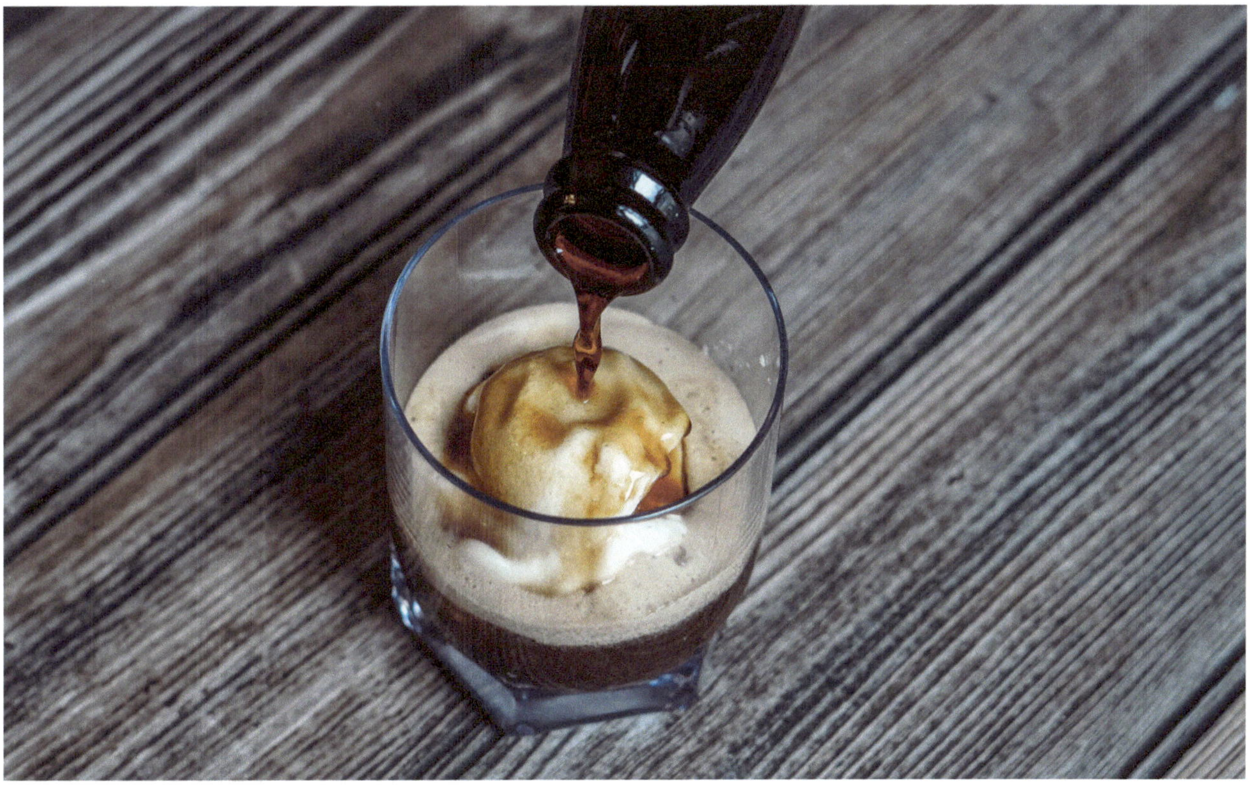

BLACK CAULDRON

MAKES 4 DESSERT/DRINK COMBOS

PAIRS WELL WITH:
- CLOSED LIQUOR STORES
- ALL NIGHTERS
- FIRESIDE CHATS

TOTAL TIME
5 MINUTES

INGREDIENTS
- 2 cups vanilla ice cream
- ¼ cup vodka
- ¼ cup fresh espresso or coffee
- 24 ounces stout beer

TIPSY TIP
If you can spring for it, something other than bottom-shelf vodka is recommended.

INSTRUCTIONS
- Grab four glasses.
- Put one scoop of ice cream into each glass.
- In a separate container, combine the vodka, beer and espresso.
- Pour the mixture over each ice cream scoop, add a spoon, and serve!

FEELING

SPORTY

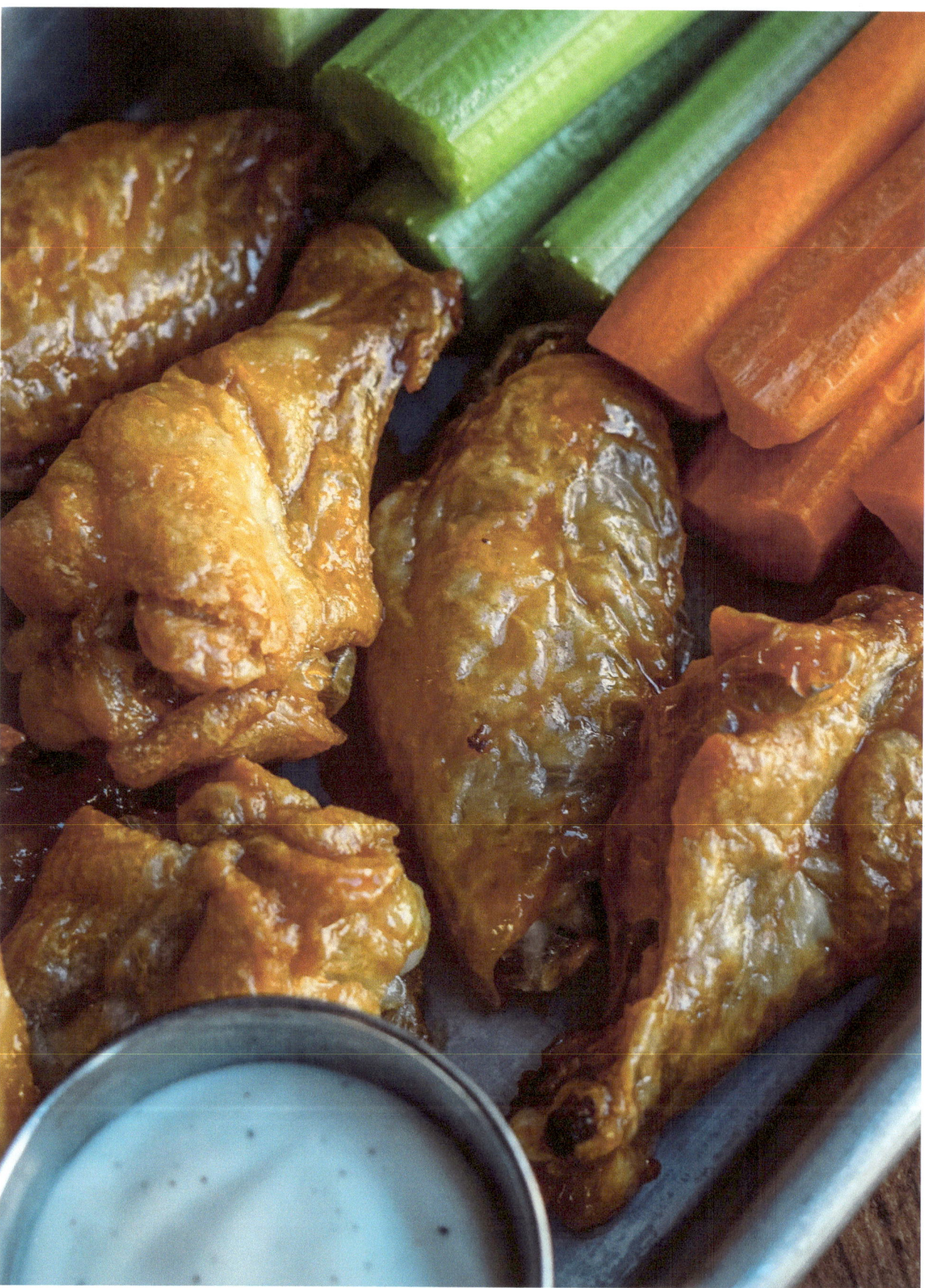

FEELING SPORTY

CRISPY BAKED CHICKEN WINGS

MAKES AN OVEN-FULL (ABOUT 8 SERVINGS)

PAIRS WELL WITH:
- BEING INTO SPORTS FOR THE SNACKS
- COLD BEER
- LOTS OF NAPKINS

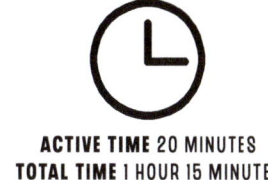

ACTIVE TIME 20 MINUTES
TOTAL TIME 1 HOUR 15 MINUTES

SPECIAL EQUIPMENT

2 baking sheets
Aluminum foil
Whisk

INGREDIENTS

5 pounds chicken wings
2 ½ Tablespoons baking powder (aluminum free)
½ teaspoon salt
Canola oil spray
Celery and carrots for garnish
Ranch or blue cheese for dipping

OPTION 1: BUFFALO SAUCE

4 Tablespoons butter, melted
½ cup hot sauce (we like Frank's)
1 Tablespoon brown sugar
½ teaspoon salt

OPTION 2: KOREAN

⅓ cup gochujang
2 Tablespoons soy sauce
1 Tablespoon rice vinegar
3 Tablespoons brown sugar
3 cloves garlic, minced
1 Tablespoon fresh ginger, grated
1 Tablespoon toasted sesame oil

HOT TIP

Baking powder with aluminum may produce a metallic taste. Check the ingredients and be sure to get it without aluminum, if possible

HERE'S THE DEAL

These wings rival the best restaurant in town.

INSTRUCTIONS

Preheat the oven to 250°F.

Reposition the oven racks so that one is in the bottom-third of the oven, and one is in the top-third.

Place the chicken on a clean, dry cutting board and pat dry with paper towels.

Cut the wings for drumettes and wingettes if you're the kind of person who cares about such things.

Place the wings into a large bowl.

Sprinkle the baking powder and salt on top and toss, making sure each piece of chicken is thoroughly covered.

Line two baking sheets with foil and spray with oil.

Place the chicken on each baking sheet, skin-side up.

Put both baking sheets on the bottom rack of the oven for 30 minutes. This helps to melt the fat under the skin to make the wings juicy.

After 30 minutes, move the pans to the top rack, increase the oven temp to 425°F, and cook for an additional 40 minutes or until golden brown. This will make the wings crisy.

While the wings are cooking, prepare your sauce of choice. For the sauces in this recipe, simply whisk the ingredients together over medium heat.

Toss the cooked wings into a bowl, add sauce, cover with a lid, and shake until fully coated.

Serve hot with carrots, celery and your salad dressing of choice.

FEELING SPORTY
SMASH BURGERS + SAUCE

MAKES 4 BURGERS

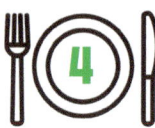

PAIRS WELL WITH:
- GAME DAY
- SMASHED POTATOES (NEXT PAGE)
- COLD BEER

ACTIVE TIME
15 MINUTES
TOTAL TIME
15 MINUTES

INGREDIENTS
BURGERS
- 1 pound 80/20 ground beef
- 1 teaspoon vegetable oil
- Salt, to taste
- 4 slices American cheese (optional)
- 4 buns

SAUCE
- ½ cup mayo
- ¼ cup ketchup
- 2 Tablespoons sweet pickle relish
- 1 teaspoon yellow mustard
- 1 ½ teaspoons sugar
- 1 ½ teaspoons white vinegar

VEG TIP
Sub plant-based meat for the ground beef for an equally epic burger.

INSTRUCTIONS
THE SAUCE
- Stir all the ingredients together and refrigerate.

THE BURGERS
- Heat a fry pan over medium-high heat.
- Add the vegetable oil to the pan, then portion the beef into four equally-sized balls
- Gently place onto the hot pan.
- Using a metal spatula or meat press, press down on each burger until it is about 1/2 inch thick. It's OK if they don't look perfectly round or have even edges!
- Season generously with salt.
- Cook for two minutes or until golden brown around the edges.
- Flip, salt to taste, and add cheese (if you like).
- Cook as desired (one minute for rare, two for medium), then remove from heat.
- Add a bun and sauce and enjoy!

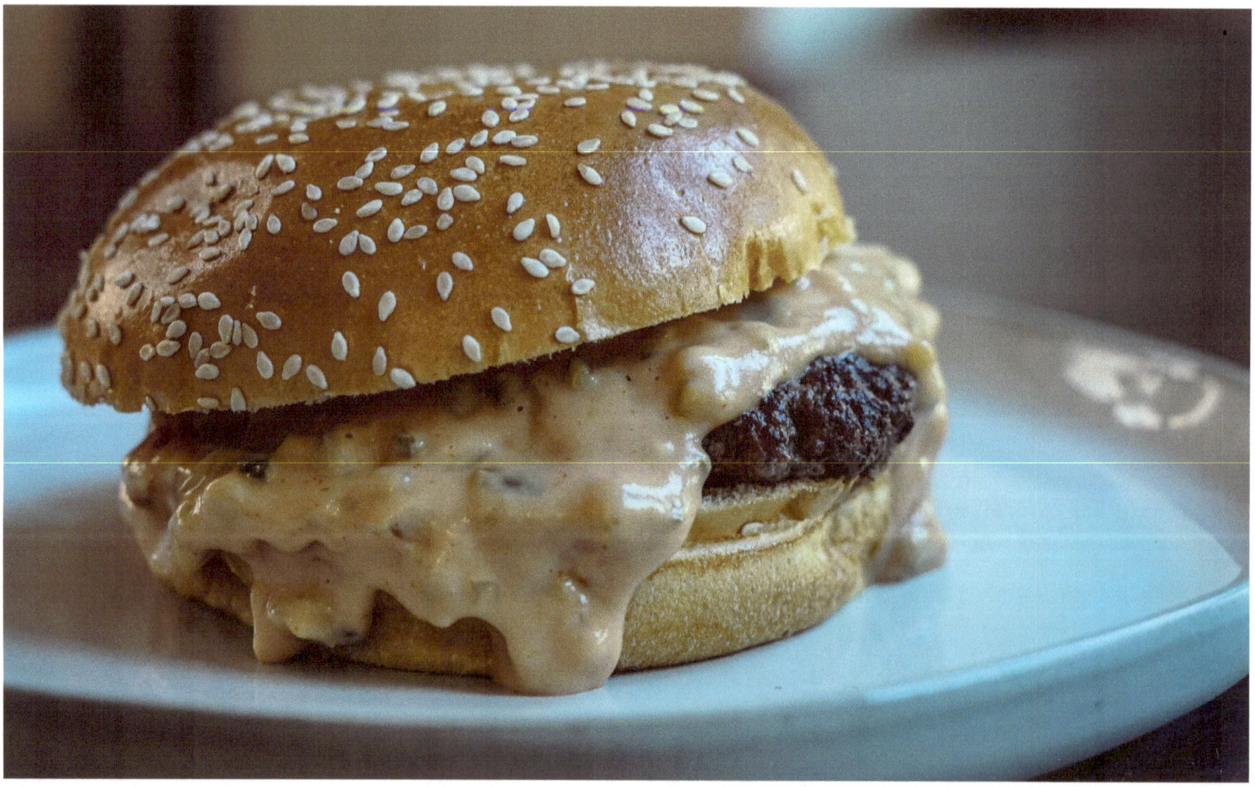

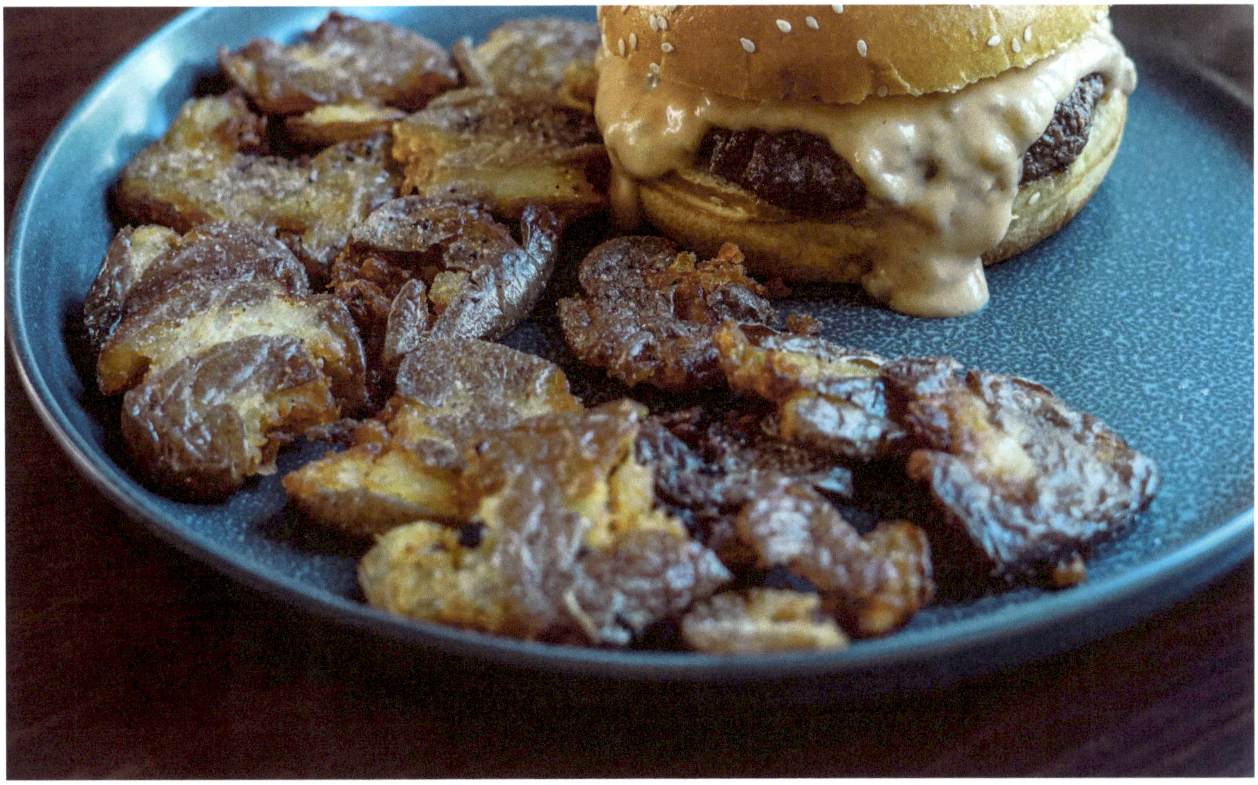

WINNING STREAK SMASHED POTATOES

MAKES 4 SERVINGS

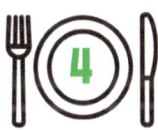

PAIRS WELL WITH:
- TATOR TOT LOYALISTS
- HEAPS OF KETCHUP
- SEASONED SALT

ACTIVE TIME
25 MINUTES
TOTAL TIME
30 MINUTES

SPECIAL EQUIPMENT
Baking sheet
Potato masher or coffee mug

INGREDIENTS
- 2 pounds small or medium potatoes (red or yellow)
- 1 cup canola oil
- Salt and pepper to taste

INSTRUCTIONS

- Toss the potatoes into a large pot, cover them with cold water, then stir in a tablespoon of salt.
- Boil until the potatoes can easily be punctured with a fork (about 15 minutes), then toss into a strainer to cool.
- Once cool enough to touch (about five minutes), "pour" the potatoes onto a baking sheet.
- Use a mug or potato masher to gently "smash" each potato until it's about as thick as a deck of cards.
- Heat the canola oil in a skillet over medium-high heat until it shines (350-375°F).
- Gently place the potatoes in the skillet, and fry until golden brown.
- Once cooked, remove the potatoes from the pan and set them on a baking sheet or large plate lined with paper towels.
- Salt and pepper to taste, then you're ready to serve!

FEELING SPORTY
BUFFALO CHEESE DIP

MAKES 1 DISH (8-10 SERVINGS)

PAIRS WELL WITH:
- KEEPING SCORE
- CRACKER VARIETY PACKS
- BIBS

PREP TIME
10 MINUTES
TOTAL TIME
30 MINUTES

GF

SPECIAL EQUIPMENT
8x8 baking dish

INGREDIENTS
- 1 can refried beans
- 1 cup hot sauce (Frank's RedHot is a classic)
- ¾ cup ranch dressing
- 1 pound canned chicken
- 8 ounces cream cheese, softened
- 1 ½ cups cheddar cheese, shredded
- Additional ½ cup shredded cheddar cheese, for topping
- 4 green onions, chopped, for topping

INSTRUCTIONS
- Start by preheating the oven to 350°F.
- Grease an 8x8 baking dish.
- Spread refried beans evenly onto the bottom of the dish.
- Mix the ingredients together, then pour evenly into the baking dish.
- Top with additional cheese and green onions, then bake until the cheese is melted (about 20 minutes).
- Turn on the broiler until the top of the dip is golden brown, but keep an eye on the oven to make sure nothing burns!
- Remove the dip from the oven and serve with anything you like - tortilla chips, celery and carrot sticks are great options. Napkins encouraged!

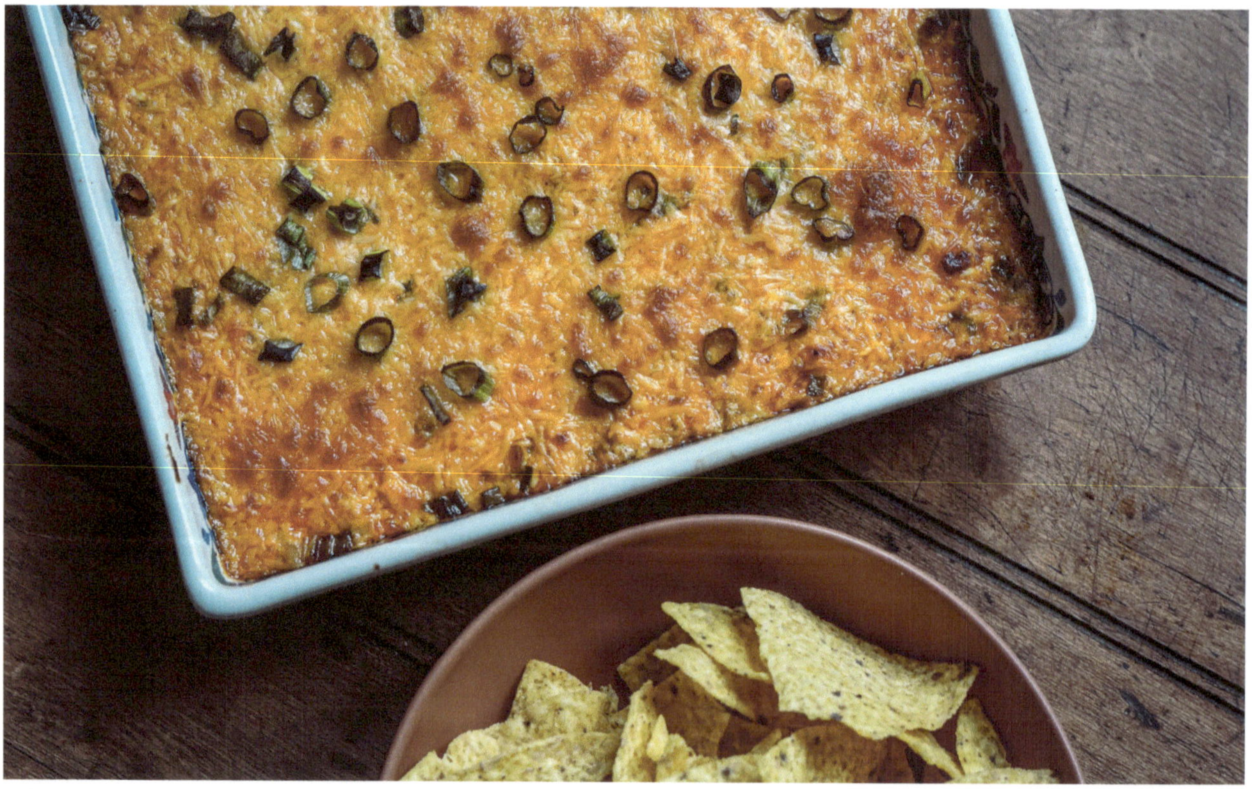

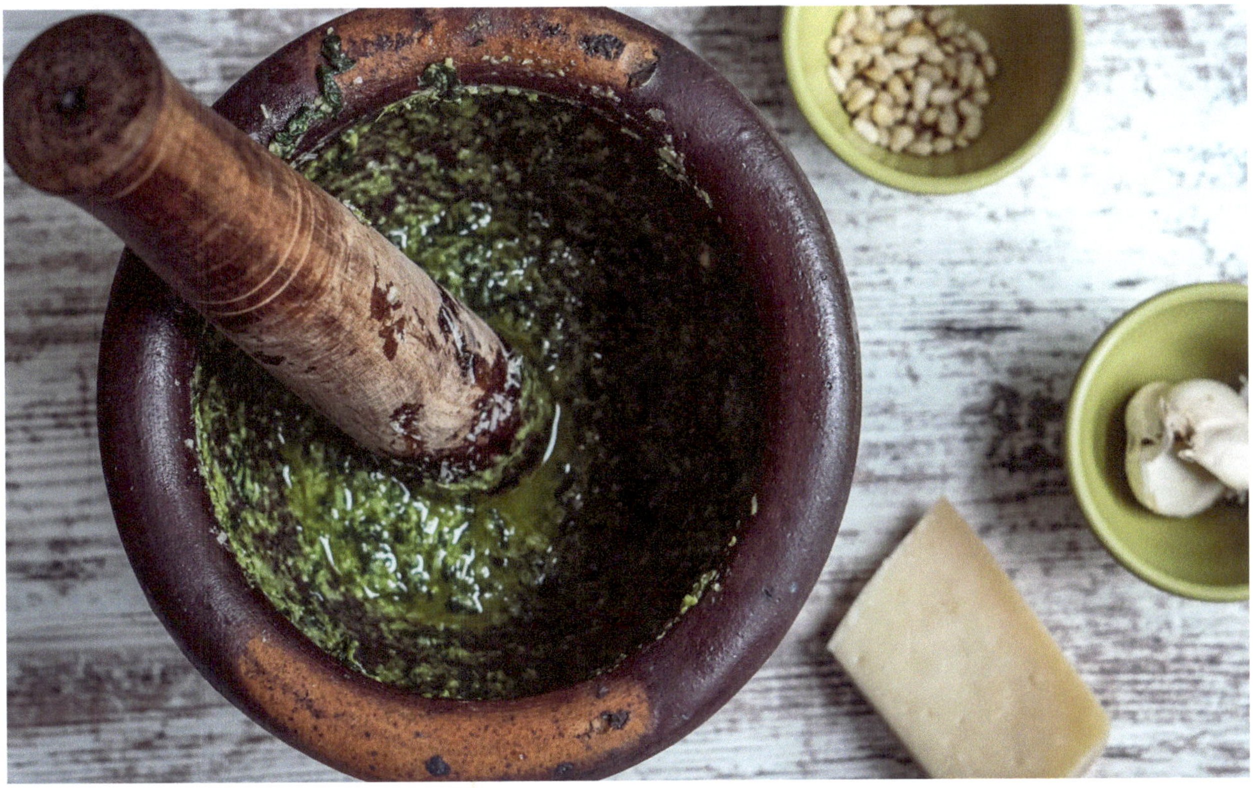

PARTY-WORTHY PESTO

MAKES 1.5 CUPS

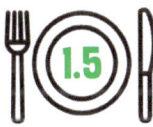

PAIRS WELL WITH:
- FRIENDS WHO WILL TELL YOU THAT YOU HAVE BASIL IN YOUR TEETH
- ELEVATING BASIC FOOD
- VEGGIE TRAYS

TOTAL TIME
20 MINUTES

SPECIAL EQUIPMENT
Mortar and pestle, food processor, or blender

INGREDIENTS
- 2 teaspoons coarse sea salt
- 2 cloves garlic, chopped
- 2 Tablespoons pine nuts or walnuts
- 4 ounces basil leaves
- 4 Tablespoons parmigiano reggiano cheese, grated
- ¾ cup olive oil, the higher quality the better

INSTRUCTIONS
- Start by combining the sea salt and garlic in the mortar and grind them together to make a thick paste.
- Add the pine nuts and continue grinding until the nuts are no longer recognizable.
- Add in the basil, a handful at a time, and continue grinding, adding in more basil when the current stuff has broken down nicely.
- Once all the basil is ground and the mixture looks like a nice paste, work in the grated cheese and olive oil until it becomes a nice, smooth sauce that resembles...well...pesto.
- Feel free to adjust the ratio of cheese, olive oil, or basil to suit your taste buds, then serve with sliced bread, veggies, pasta, or a spoon.

LARGE-BATCH TIP
Walnuts can be used as a cheaper and easier-to-find alternative to pine nuts.

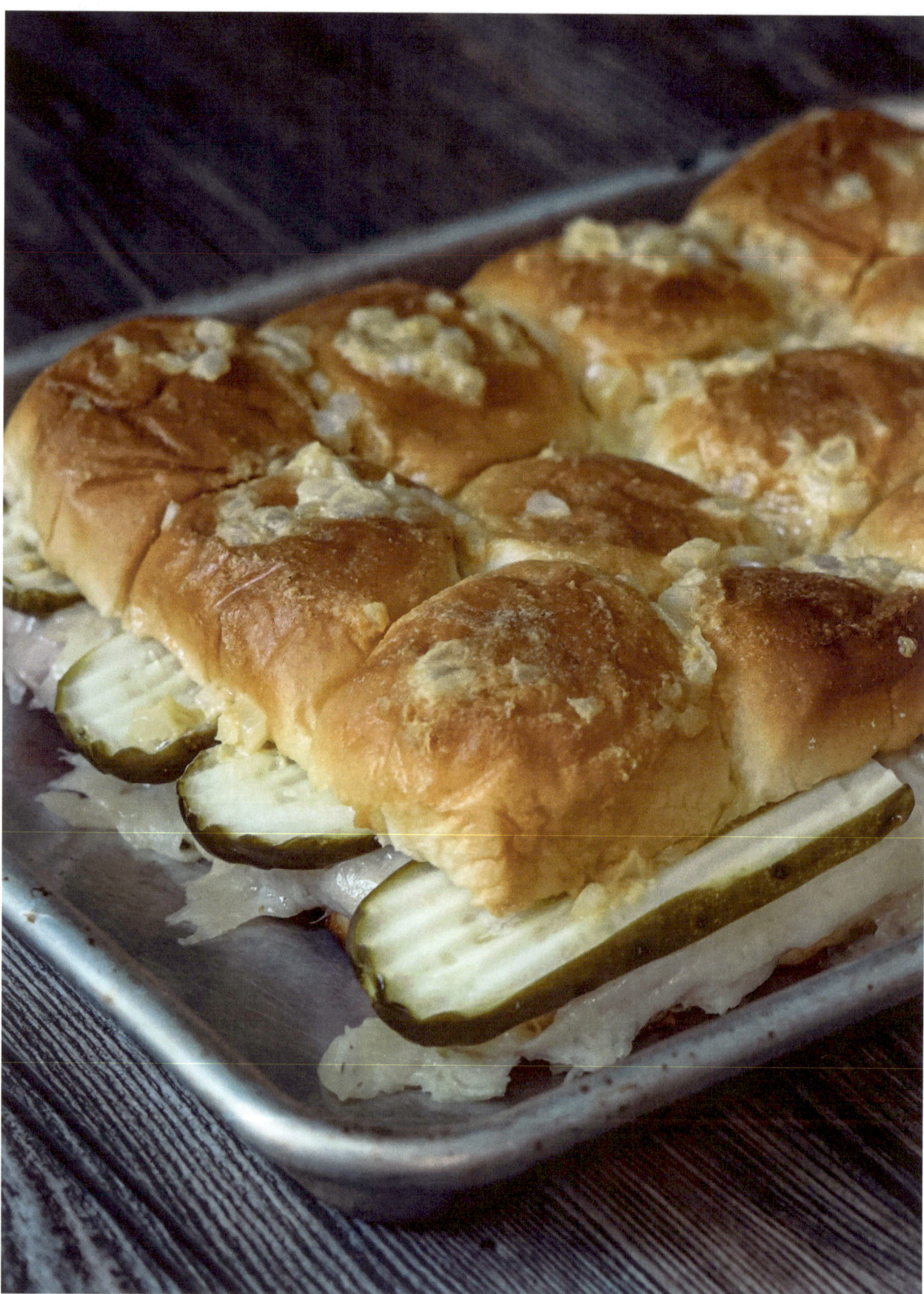

FEELING SPORTY

(ALMOST) CUBAN SLIDERS

MAKES 12 SLIDERS

PAIRS WELL WITH:
- THE FRIEND WHO ALWAYS BRINGS CHIPS
- GRAZING
- BEER PUNCH (NEXT PAGE)

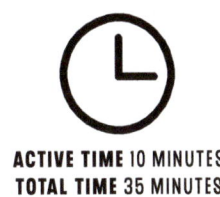

ACTIVE TIME 10 MINUTES
TOTAL TIME 35 MINUTES

SPECIAL EQUIPMENT

Baking sheet
Aluminum foil

INGREDIENTS

1 pack Hawaiian sweet rolls (usually 12 rolls)
¼ pound sliced deli ham (8-12 slices)
8-12 slices swiss cheese
2 cups dill pickles slices
4 Tablespoons melted butter
¼ cup onion, diced
2 Tablespoons dijon mustard

HERE'S THE DEAL

Like cubans and love sliders? We got you.
For a little extra pizzazz (and a more traditional cubano flavor), feel free to add pulled pork to this recipe (see the Korean Pulled Pork recipe in Adventurous).

INSTRUCTIONS

Preheat the oven to 350°F.

Cut the rolls into two halves (you can keep the individual rolls stuck together as you do this).

Set the top half of the rolls aside.

Lay the ham evenly across the bottom half of the rolls, then follow with the cheese and pickles.

Melt the butter in a small saucepan.

Once the butter is fully melted, add the onion and cook until it is soft and slightly translucent.

Stir in the dijon mustard, then spread about half of the butter mixture onto the underside of bun tops.

Place the tops onto the bottoms to "close" the sandwich, then take the remaining butter mixture and spread it evenly across the bun tops.

Place the whole thing on a baking sheet and cover with foil.

Bake in the oven for 15 minutes, then pull the foil off and continue baking for another 10 minutes, until the buns are nicely toasted.

Pull out of the oven and let the sliders rest for a few minutes before serving.

FEELING SPORTY

MVP BEER PUNCH

MAKES 4+ DRINKS

PAIRS WELL WITH:
- FOLDING CHAIRS
- ZERO PTO
- CHIPS & DIP

TOTAL TIME
2 MINUTES

EQUIPMENT
Pitcher, large bowl, or bucket

INGREDIENTS
- 3 light beers (dark beers don't play nicely with this recipe)
- 2 cups pineapple juice
- 2 cups ginger ale
- Fresh pineapple, for garnish

INSTRUCTIONS
- Pour the liquid ingredients into a pitcher or large bowl.
- Gently stir.
- Serve garnished with pineapple, or, if you want to be a show-off, serve inside the pineapple.

N/A TIP
Swap in N/A beer (Athletic is our favorite) for beer flavor without the buzz.

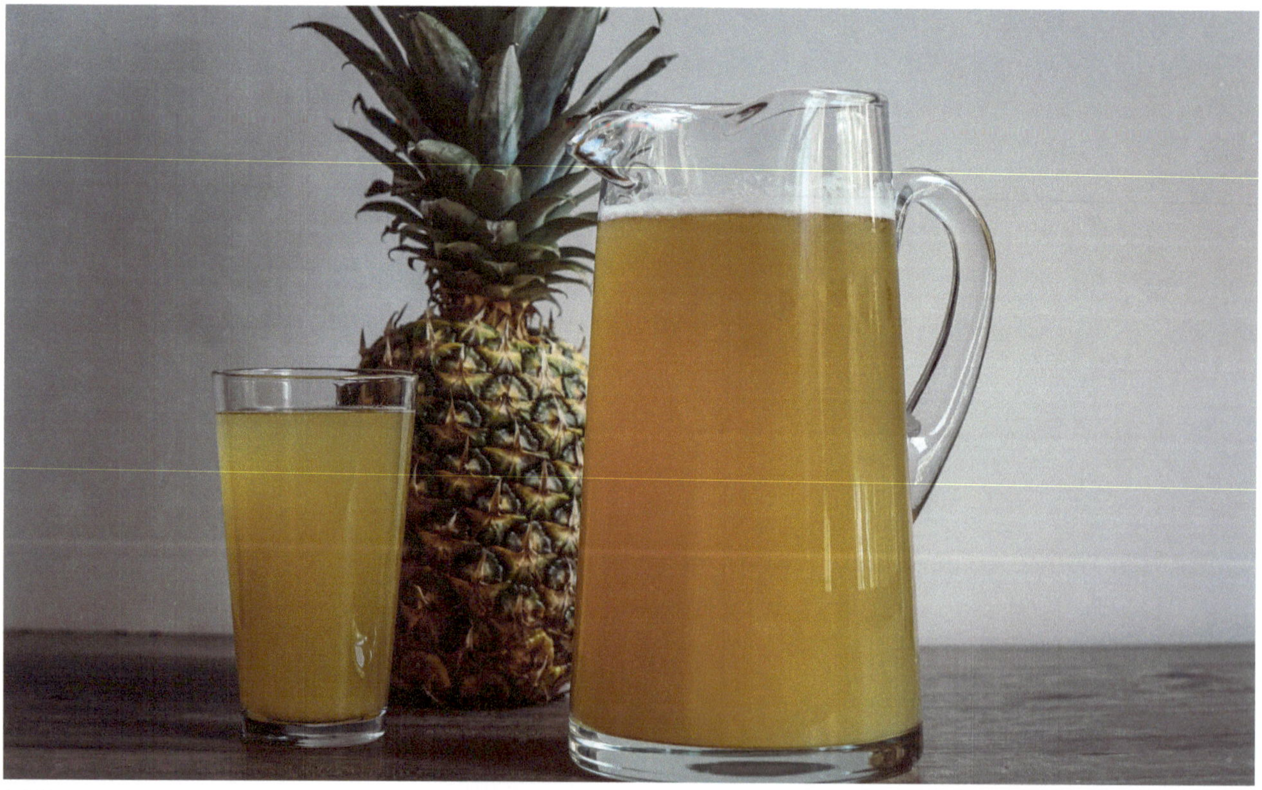

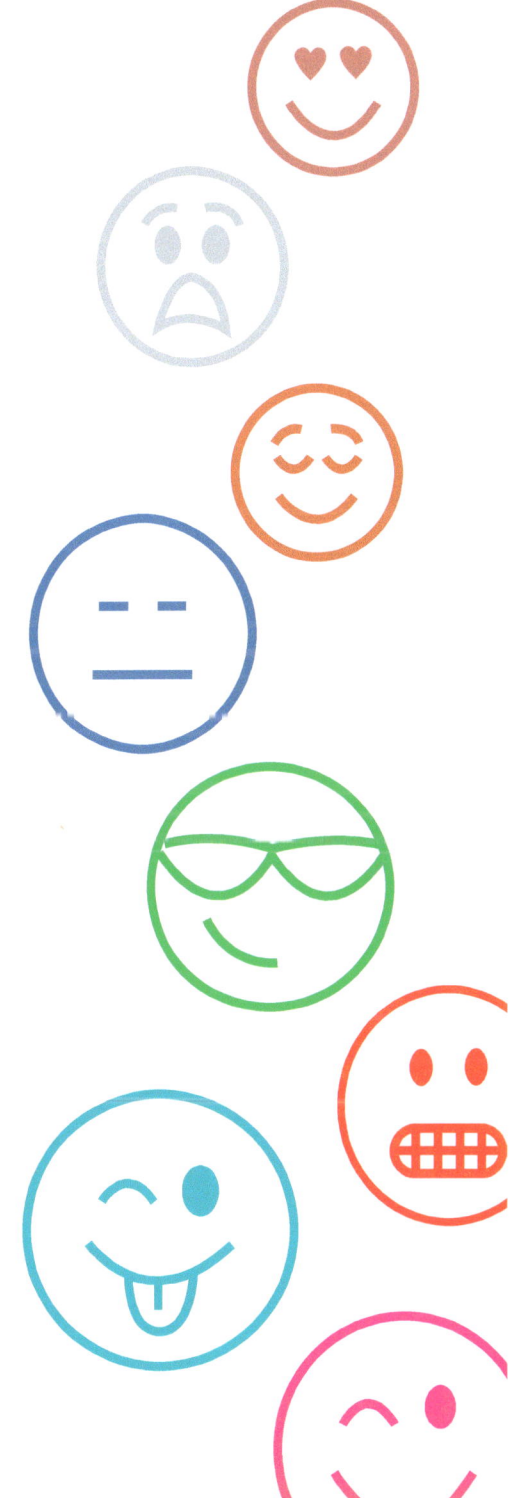

INDEX

A

aioli
38
almond
31, 82
amaro
90
aperol
90
apple
29, 31, 50, 112
apricot
117
avocado
5, 29, 32, 79, 82, 86, 93, 118, 129

B

bacon
65, 79
basil
11, 41, 61, 86, 105, 140
beans
25, 58, 118, 139
beef
30, 58, 59, 101, 137
beer
132, 136, 137, 142, 143
biscuit
50, 64
bitters
67, 68
blueberries
51
bourbon
46, 67, 89, 90, 109, 111, 112
brandy
112, 130
bread
11, 40, 41, 43, 50, 54, 58, 59, 61, 96, 100, 117, 119, 126, 129, 140
buns
4, 40, 137, 142
butter
14, 39, 40, 45, 50, 51, 54, 55, 64, 65, 78, 83, 86, 87, 96, 97, 104, 108, 109, 128, 136, 142
buttercream
109
butterscotch
60

C

cabbage
93
cake
109, 122
carrot
4, 26, 55, 59, 136, 139
cauliflower
38
celery
4, 26, 55, 59, 136, 139
champagne
131
cheese
8, 25, 29, 30, 40, 54, 58, 61, 71, 86, 96, 101, 104, 105, 117, 128, 136, 137, 139, 140, 142
chicken
4, 10, 14, 15, 18, 19, 26, 30, 54, 55, 64, 75, 105, 136, 139
chives
54, 79
cilantro
10, 14, 19, 25, 27, 32, 58, 79, 93, 100, 118
cinnamon
9, 50, 51, 112
cocktail
20, 21, 22, 46, 66, 68, 89, 90, 113, 131
cocoa
39, 71, 109
coconut
10, 14, 31, 45, 55, 64, 75, 82, 83, 105, 109
coffee
50, 71, 78, 104, 132
cookies
39, 71, 97, 114
cornbread
58
cream
30, 42, 58, 61, 65, 75, 83, 96, 101, 104, 105, 114, 139

E

eggs
8, 11, 25, 35, 36, 51, 55, 58, 71, 78, 79, 83, 87, 97, 100, 104, 108, 109, 122

F

fennel
74
flour
18, 43, 51, 55, 64, 78, 93, 96, 97, 100, 101, 104, 108, 109

G

garlic
4, 10, 11, 14, 15, 18, 26, 38, 54, 58, 59, 64, 74, 75, 82, 86, 93, 100,

105, 119, 123, 125, 126, 128, 129, 136, 140
ginger
 15, 18, 66, 112, 119, 130, 136, 143
gnocchi
 86, 123
goat (cheese)
 8, 29, 117
gochujang
 4, 136
gruyere
 54, 96
guacamole
 101, 129

H

hashbrowns
 51
hollandaise
 87

J

jalapeno
 93

K

kale
 27, 29, 119

L

lemon
 15, 18, 21, 29, 32, 46, 66, 68, 74, 75, 79, 82, 87, 89, 90, 100, 113, 131
lemongrass
 10, 18
lime
 10, 14, 19, 20, 22, 27, 93, 118

M

mascarpone
 71
mayo
 5, 38, 61, 79, 100, 137
milk
 10, 14, 30, 39, 42, 51, 55, 58, 64, 78, 82, 97, 104, 108, 109, 114
mozzarella
 128
muffins
 78, 87
mustard
 4, 29, 38, 79, 96, 137, 142

N

noodles
 26, 35, 96

O

oats
 39
onion
 4, 5, 8, 9, 14, 19, 25, 30, 32, 35, 54, 55, 58, 59, 64, 65, 75, 100, 104, 119, 125, 139, 142
orange
 15, 67, 108, 112, 125, 130
oregano
 58, 64, 75, 82, 93, 105

P

pancetta
 11
parmesan
 40, 75, 86, 105, 123
peanuts
 14, 27, 119
pineapple
 22, 93, 118, 122, 143
pizza
 43
potato
 26, 51, 59, 65, 74, 75, 137, 138

R

raspberries
 78
rum
 112

S

sage
 8, 74, 125
salmon
 82, 87, 100
salsa
 22, 25, 101, 118
sausage
 8, 64, 75, 108
scallions
 104
scallops
 86
scotch
 66

146

T

tahini
 35
tequila
 20, 22
tomato
 11, 41, 58, 59, 61, 82, 86, 87, 101, 105, 119

V

vanilla
 31, 39, 51, 60, 78, 83, 97, 109, 114

vodka
 18, 132

W

walnuts
 123, 140
wings
 18, 136

Y

yeast
 43
yogurt
 15, 93

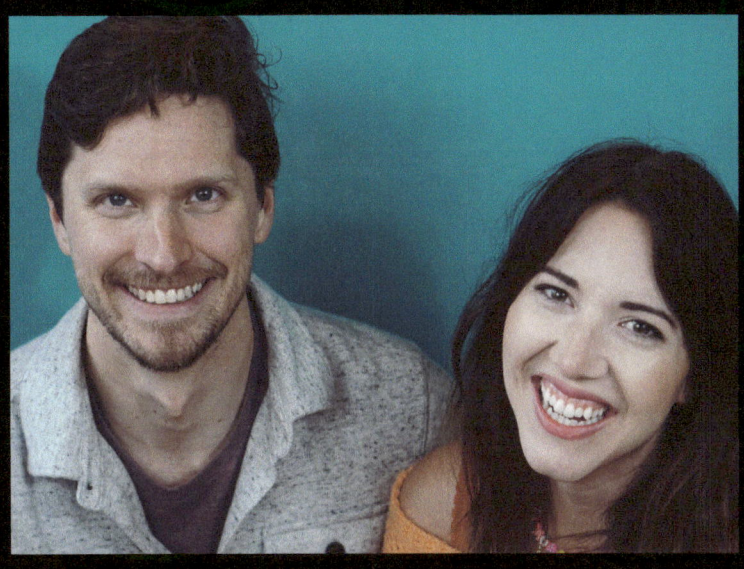

ABOUT THE AUTHORS

Rob Murray is a home-grown chef. He has refined his craft through simple trial and error, food-snob-friends' recommendations, and YouTube tutorials, among many things.

Niki Murray is a wordsmith and master dabbler who has the pleasure of eating Rob's food.

Rob and Niki currently reside in Minnesota, where Cozy is not only a mood, but a lifestyle.

MOOD FOOD

www.ingramcontent.com/pod-product-compliance
Lightning Source LLC
Chambersburg PA
CBHW041423010526
44119CB00015B/349